The Social Neuroscience of Empathy

Social Neuroscience Series
Series Editors John T. Cacioppo and Gary G. Berntson
Series Editorial Board Ralph Adolphs, C. Sue Carter, Richard J. Davidson,
Martha K. McClintock, Bruce S. McEwen, Michael J. Meaney, Daniel L. Schacter,
Esther M. Sternberg, Steve S. Suomi, and Shelley E. Taylor

Foundations in Social Neuroscience
edited by John T. Cacioppo, Gary G. Berntson, Ralph Adolphs, C. Sue Carter, Richard J. Davidson,
Martha K. McClintock, Bruce S. McEwen, Michael J. Meaney, Daniel L. Schacter, Esther M. Sternberg,
Steve S. Suomi, and Shelley E. Taylor

Essays in Social Neuroscience
edited by John T. Cacioppo and Gary G. Berntson

Social Neuroscience: People Thinking about Thinking People
edited by John T. Cacioppo, Penny S. Visser, and Cynthia L. Pickett

The Social Neuroscience of Empathy
edited by Jean Decety and William Ickes

The Social Neuroscience of Empathy

edited by Jean Decety and William Ickes

A Bradford Book
The MIT Press
Cambridge, Massachusetts
London, England

For information about special quantity discounts, please e-mail special_sales@mitpress.mit.edu

This book was set in Stone Sans and Stone Serif by SNP Best-set Typesetter Ltd., Hong Kong. Printed and bound in the United States of America.

Library of Congress Cataloging-in-Publication Data

The social neuroscience of empathy / edited by Jean Decety and William Ickes.
     p.   cm.—(Social neuroscience)
"A Bradford book."
Includes bibliographical references and index.
ISBN 978-0-262-01297-3 (hardcover : alk. paper) 1. Empathy. 2. Neurosciences. 3. Social psychology. I. Decety, Jean. II. Ickes, William John.
BF575.E55S63   2009
155.2′32—dc22
                                                                                          2008034814

10 9 8 7 6 5 4 3 2

Contents

Introduction: Seeking to Understand the Minds (and Brains) of People Who Are Seeking to Understand Other People's Minds

After decades as the cultivated interest of scholars in philosophy and in clinical and developmental psychology, empathy research is suddenly everywhere! Seemingly overnight it has blossomed into a vibrant, multidisciplinary field of study and has crossed the boundaries of clinical and developmental psychology to plant its roots firmly in the soil of personality and social psychology, mainstream cognitive psychology, and cognitive-affective neuroscience.

To account for the recent explosion of empathy research, we must trace its growth to roots that are less obvious but even deeper than those mentioned so far: the study of the capacity for empathy in evolutionary biology and evolutionary psychology. As Sue Carter, James Harris, and Stephen Porges argue in chapter 13 of the present volume, the capacity for empathy in humans and their progenitor species developed over millions of years of evolutionary history, in ways that are only now becoming clear. Although it is impossible to travel back in time and observe these developments directly, the evidence for them is available in the neuroanatomical continuities and differences that can be observed across the phylogenetic spectrum.

Given the long evolutionary history of the capacity for empathy, there is some irony in the fact that the word *empathy* has a relatively short history, being not much more than a hundred years old (see Ickes, 2003, chap. 4). Not only is empathy a rather recent construct, but it is a complicated one that, from its very introduction, has been used by different writers in very different ways.

It is appropriate, therefore, that an interdisciplinary book such as this one begin with a critical examination of the concept of empathy and the range of different meanings it has acquired to date. Accordingly, in chapter 1 Daniel Batson examines eight conceptually distinct phenomena that have all been labeled "empathy" and calls for a more theoretically coherent articulation of this important construct.

The second part of this volume vividly illustrates the divergent views of empathy that Batson has noted by presenting empathy variously as emotional contagion based on unconscious mimicry (chapters 2 and 3); as the projection of one's own thoughts and feelings onto others (chapter 4); as the ability to accurately infer another person's thoughts and feelings (chapter 5); as a complex affective-inferential process that often translates into prosocial behavior (chapter 6); and as a fundamental aspect of social development that contemporary educators should urgently promote (chapter 7).

The third part of this volume offers a range of clinical perspectives on empathy. It begins with a review of the role of empathy in the Rogerian client-centered perspective (chapter 8), continues with a dialogical view of how empathy is achieved during psychotherapy (chapter 9); then explores the concept of empathic resonance from a neuroscience perspective (chapter 10); links empathy to the study of morality and social convention (chapter 11); and examines the role of empathy in people's reactions to others in pain (chapter 12).

The fourth and final part of this volume explores the deepest and oldest roots of empathy by examining its evolutionary history and its neuroanatomical history. Chapter 13 provides an evolutionary view of empathy that focuses on how emotional and visceral states influence how we feel about and react to others and thus affect our capacity for empathy. Chapter 14 focuses more specifically on the mirror neuron system, arguing that it provides a neural and behavioral foundation for interpersonal understanding. Chapter 15 shows how recent work in the area of cognitive-affective neuroscience has enabled researchers to identify a clear distinction between empathy and personal distress in terms of the different neural substrates that underlie the two phenomena. Finally, Chapter 16, noting the deficits in empathic behavior that are observed following brain damage, proposes that empathy involves separate, albeit interacting, brain networks.

The new discipline of social neuroscience is exciting because it integrates, builds upon, and challenges more traditional approaches. For example, theories in social psychology provide important guidelines for investigating the information-processing mechanisms that underlie empathy and determine their neural instantiation. The social neuroscience approach can also help to disambiguate competing social theories; in the domain of empathy; for instance, this approach has been used to validate at a neurological level the distinction between personal distress and empathic concern. Finally, the social neuroscience approach has led some theorists to challenge existing beliefs—for example, the notion that there are domain-specific "theory of mind" modules in the brain. Alternative accounts (Decety & Lamm, 2007; Stone & Gerrans, 2007) argue that (a) elementary computational operations have evolved to perform social functions, and (b) evolution has constructed layers of increasing complexity, from nonrepresentational to representational and meta-representational mechanisms, which may be sufficient to provide a complete understanding of human social cognition.

The present book is not, and cannot be, the final word on empathy research. It does, however, seek to provide the reader with a representative sampling of current, state-of-the-art knowledge about empathy—knowledge that draws from contemporary work in biology, developmental psychology, cognitive-affective neuroscience and neuropsychology, social and cognitive psychology, and the more applied disciplines of clinical and health psychology.

A hallmark of the newest of these disciplines, the emerging field of social neuroscience, is its use of methods that bridge a variety of disciplines and levels of analysis. We hope that the reader will, like us, be excited by the potential for cross-disciplinary integration that the study of social neuroscience promises. We also hope that the chapters in this book will stimulate even more sharing of ideas and collaboration in research between the different academic domains that actively pursue the study of empathy.

References

Decety, J., & Lamm, C. (2007). The role of the right temporoparietal junction in social interaction: How low-level computational processes contribute to meta-cognition. *Neuroscientist, 13,* 580–593.

Ickes, W. (2003). *Everyday mind reading: Understanding what other people think and feel.* Amherst, NY: Prometheus Books.

Stone, V. E., & Gerrans, P. (2007). What's domain-specific about theory of mind. *Social Neuroscience, 1* (2–4), 309–319.

The Social Neuroscience of Empathy

I What Is Empathy?

1 These Things Called Empathy: Eight Related but Distinct Phenomena

C. Daniel Batson

Students of empathy can seem a cantankerous lot. Although they typically agree that empathy is important, they often disagree about why it is important, about what effects it has, about where it comes from, and even about what it is. The term *empathy* is currently applied to more than a half-dozen phenomena. These phenomena are related to one another, but they are not elements, aspects, facets, or components of a single thing that is empathy, as one might say that an attitude has cognitive, affective, and behavioral components. Rather, each is a conceptually distinct, stand-alone psychological state. Further, each of these states has been called by names other than empathy. Opportunities for disagreement abound.

In an attempt to sort out this disagreement, I wish first to identify two distinct questions that empathy is thought to answer. Then I wish to identify eight distinct phenomena that have been called empathy. Finally, I wish to relate these eight phenomena to the two questions.[1]

Empathy as an Answer to Two Different Questions

Application of the term *empathy* to so many distinct phenomena is, in part, a result of researchers invoking empathy to provide an answer to two quite different questions: How can one know what another person is thinking and feeling? What leads one person to respond with sensitivity and care to the suffering of another? For some students of empathy, answers to these two questions are related. However, many more seek to answer the first question without concern to answer the second, or vice versa.

The first question has been of particular interest to philosophers, cognitive scientists, neurophysiologists, primatologists, and developmental psychologists interested in the theory of mind. Both *theory theorists*, who suggest that we use our lay theories about the mind to infer the internal states of others, and *simulation theorists*, who suggest that we imagine ourselves in others' situations and read their internal states from our own, have invoked empathy to explain how we humans come to know what others are thinking and feeling.

The question of what leads us to respond with sensitive care to another's suffering has been of particular interest to philosophers and to developmental and social psychologists seeking to understand and promote prosocial action. The goal of these researchers is not to explain a particular form of knowledge but to explain a particular form of action: action by one person that effectively addresses the need of another. Those using empathy to answer this question are apt to say that empathic feelings *for* the other—feelings of sympathy, compassion, tenderness, and the like—produce motivation to relieve the suffering of the person for whom empathy is felt.

Eight Uses of the Term *Empathy*

An example may help clarify distinctions among different uses of the term *empathy*. Imagine that you meet a friend for lunch. She seems distracted, staring into space, not very talkative, a bit down. Gradually, she begins to speak, then to cry. She explains that she just learned that she is losing her job because of downsizing. She says that she is not angry but that she is hurt, and a bit scared. You feel very sorry for her, and say so. You are also reminded that there has been talk of job cuts where you work as well. Seeing your friend so upset makes you feel a bit anxious and uneasy. You also feel a brief flash of relief—"Thank God it wasn't me!" At least eight different psychological states you might experience in this interchange correspond to distinct concepts of empathy.

Concept 1: Knowing Another Person's Internal State, Including His or Her Thoughts and Feelings

Some clinicians and researchers have called knowing another person's internal state empathy (e.g., Preston & de Waal, 2002; Wispé, 1986). Others have called this knowledge "cognitive empathy" (Eslinger, 1998; Zahn-Waxler, Robinson, & Emde, 1992) or "empathic accuracy" (Ickes, 1993).

Sometimes, to ascertain what someone else is thinking and feeling can pose quite a problem, especially when one has only limited clues. But in our example, knowing your friend's internal state is relatively easy. Once she explains, you may be confident that you know what is on her mind: losing her job. From what she says, and perhaps even more from the way she acts, you may also think you know how she feels: she is hurt and scared. Of course, you could be wrong, at least about some nuances and details.

Concept 2: Adopting the Posture or Matching the Neural Responses of an Observed Other

Adopting the posture or expression of an observed other is a definition of empathy in many dictionaries. The philosopher Gordon (1995) speaks of this as "facial empathy." Among psychologists, adopting another's posture is more likely to be called "motor mimicry" (Dimberg, Thunberg, & Elmehed, 2000; Hoffman, 2000) or "imitation" (Lipps, 1903; Meltzoff & Moore, 1997; Titchener, 1909).

Preston and de Waal (2002) proposed what they claim is a unified theory of empathy that focuses on mimicked neural representations rather than mimicked motor activity. Their theory is based on a perception-action model. According to this model, perceiving another in a given situation automatically leads one to match the other's neural state because perception and action rely in part on the same neural circuits. As a result of the matched neural representation, which need not produce either matched motor activity or awareness, one comes to feel something of what the other feels, and thereby to understand the other's internal state.

To claim that either neural response matching or motor mimicry is the unifying source of all empathic feelings seems to be an overestimation of their role, especially among humans. Perceptual neural representations do not always and automatically lead to feelings, whether matched or unmatched. And at a motor level, neither humans nor other species mimic all actions of others. To find oneself tensing and twisting when watching someone balance on a tightrope is a familiar experience; it is hard to resist. Yet we may watch someone file papers with little inclination to mimic the action. Something more than automatic mimicry must be involved to select those actions that are mimicked and those that are not. Moreover, it has been found that mimicry itself may not be as reactive and automatic as has been assumed. Meltzoff and Moore (1997) present much evidence that mimicry or imitation is an active, goal-directed process even in infants. And in adults, mimicry often serves a higher-order communicative function (LaFrance & Ickes, 1981). In the words of Bavelas and colleagues (1986), "I show how you feel" in order to convey "fellow feeling" or support.

Rather than relying solely on response matching or mimicry to provide clues to the internal states of others, humans can also use memory and general knowledge to infer what others think and feel in various situations (Singer et al., 2004; Tomasello, 1999). Indeed, the problem of anthropomorphism arises precisely because we humans have the ability—and inclination—to make such inferences, even about other species. Equally important, humans can rely on direct communication from one another to learn about internal states. In our example, your friend told you what she was thinking and feeling.

Concept 3: Coming to Feel as Another Person Feels

Coming to feel the same emotion that another person feels is another common dictionary definition of empathy. It is also a definition used by some philosophers (e.g., Darwall, 1998; Sober & Wilson, 1998), neuroscientists (Damasio, 2003; Decety & Chaminade, 2003; Eslinger, 1998), and psychologists (Eisenberg & Strayer, 1987; Preston & de Waal, 2002). Often, those who use this definition qualify it by saying that the empathizer need not feel exactly the same emotion, only a similar one (e.g., Hoffman, 2000). However, what determines whether an emotion is similar enough is never made clear.

Key to this use of the term empathy is not only emotion matching but also emotion "catching" (Hatfield, Cacioppo, & Rapson, 1994). To know that one person has come to feel as another feels, it is necessary to know more than that the former has a physiological response of roughly the same magnitude at roughly the same time as the latter—what

Levenson and Ruef (1992) called "shared physiology." Shared physiology provides no clear evidence of either matching (the observer's arousal might be associated with a qualitatively different emotion) or catching (rather than being a response to the target's emotional state, the observer's arousal might be a parallel response to a shared situation, perhaps one to which the target's response drew attention).

Among philosophers, coming to feel as the other feels has often been called "sympathy," not empathy (Hume, 1740/1896; Smith, 1759/1853). Among psychologists, it has been called "emotional contagion" (Hatfield, Cacioppo, & Rapson, 1994), "affective empathy" (Zahn-Waxler, Robinson, & Emde, 1992), and "automatic emotional empathy" (Hodges & Wegner, 1997).

In one of the most frequently cited studies of the developmental origins of empathy, Sagi and Hoffman (1976) presented one- to two-day-old infants either with tape-recorded sounds of another infant crying, with sounds of a synthetic nonhuman cry, or with no sounds. Those infants presented with another infant's cry cried significantly more than those presented with a synthetic cry or with silence. Sagi and Hoffman (1976, p. 176), and many others since, interpreted this difference as evidence of an inborn "rudimentary empathic distress reaction," that is, as evidence of one newborn infant catching and matching another's affective state.

However, to interpret this research as evidence of an inborn rudimentary empathic reaction seems premature. There are alternative explanations for crying in response to another infant's cry, alternatives that to my knowledge have never been recognized in the literature. To give but one example, crying in response to another infant's cry may be a competitive response that increases the chances of getting food or comfort. (The infants in the Sagi and Hoffman study were tested 1 to 1½ hours before feeding time.) Imagine that we did a similar study using baby birds in a nest. We would not likely interpret the rapid spread of peeping and open-mouth straining once one baby bird starts peeping and straining as a rudimentary empathic reaction.

Concept 4: Intuiting or Projecting Oneself into Another's Situation
Listening to your friend, you might have asked yourself what it would be like to be a young woman just told she is losing her job. Imaginatively projecting oneself into another's situation is the psychological state referred to by Lipps (1903) as *Einfühlung* and for which Titchener (1909) first coined the English word *empathy*. Both were intrigued by the process whereby a writer or painter imagines what it would be like to be some specific person or some inanimate object, such as a gnarled, dead tree on a windswept hillside.

This original definition of empathy as aesthetic projection often appears in dictionaries, and it has appeared in recent philosophical discussions of simulation as an alternative to *theory theories* of mind. But such projection is rarely what is meant by empathy in contemporary psychology. Still, Wispé (1968) included such projection in his analysis of sympathy and empathy, calling it "aesthetic empathy."

Concept 5: Imagining How Another Is Thinking and Feeling

Rather than imagine how it would feel to be a young woman just told she is losing her job, you might imagine how your friend is thinking and feeling. Your imagining can be based both on what she says and does and on your knowledge of her character, values, and desires. Stotland (1969) spoke of this as a particular form of perspective taking, an "imagine him" perspective. More generally, it has been called an "imagine other" perspective (Batson, 1991).

Wispé (1968) called imagining how another is feeling "psychological empathy" to differentiate it from the aesthetic empathy of concept 4. Adolphs (1999) called it "empathy" or "projection"; Ruby and Decety (2004) called it "empathy" or "perspective taking."

In a perceptive analysis from a therapeutic perspective, Barrett-Lennard (1981) spoke of adopting an "empathic attentional set." This set involves "a process of feeling into, in which Person A opens him- or herself in a deeply responsive way to Person B's feelings and experiencing but without losing awareness that B is a distinct other self" (p. 92). At issue is not so much what one knows about the feelings and thoughts of the other but one's sensitivity to the way the other is affected by his or her situation.

Concept 6: Imagining How One Would Think and Feel in the Other's Place

Adam Smith (1759/1853) colorfully referred to the act of imagining how one would think and feel in another person's situation as "changing places in fancy." Mead (1934) sometimes called it "role taking" and sometimes "empathy"; Povinelli (1993) called it "cognitive empathy." Darwall (1998) spoke of "projective empathy" or "simulation." In the Piagetian tradition, imagining how one would think in the other's place has been called either "perspective taking" or "decentering" (Piaget, 1953).

Stotland (1969) called this an "imagine-self" perspective, distinguishing it from the imagine-other perspective of concept 5. The imagine-other and imagine-self forms of perspective taking have often been confused or equated with one another, despite empirical evidence suggesting that they should not be (Batson, Early, & Salvarani, 1997; Stotland, 1969).

To adopt an imagine-self perspective is in some ways similar to the act of projecting oneself into another's situation (concept 4). Yet these two concepts were developed independently in very different contexts, one aesthetic and the other interpersonal, and the self remains more focal here than in aesthetic projection, so it seems best to keep them separate.

Concept 7: Feeling Distress at Witnessing Another Person's Suffering

A state of distress evoked by witnessing another's distress—your feelings of anxiety and unease evoked by seeing how upset your friend was—has been given a variety of names, including "empathy" (Krebs, 1975), "empathic distress" (Hoffman, 1981), and "personal distress" (Batson, 1991).

This state does not involve feeling distressed *for* the other (see concept 8) or distressed *as* the other (concept 3). It involves feeling distressed *by* the state of the other.

Concept 8: Feeling for Another Person Who Is Suffering

In contemporary social psychology, the term "empathy" or "empathic concern" has often been used to refer to an other-oriented emotional response elicited by and congruent with the perceived welfare of someone else (e.g., Batson, 1991). *Other-oriented* here refers to the focus of the emotion; it is felt *for* the other. *Congruent* refers to the valence of the emotion—positive when the perceived welfare of the other is positive, negative when the perceived welfare is negative. To speak of congruence does not imply that the content of the emotion is the same or even similar, as in concept 3. You might, for example, feel sad or sorry for your friend, who is scared and upset.

Other-oriented emotion felt when another is perceived to be in need has not always been called empathy. It has also been called "pity" or "compassion" (Hume, 1740/1896; Smith, 1759/1853), "sympathetic distress" (Hoffman, 1981, 2000), and simply "sympathy" (Darwall, 1998; Eisenberg & Strayer, 1987; Preston & de Waal, 2002; Sober & Wilson, 1998; Wispé, 1986).

Implications

I have listed these eight phenomena to which the term empathy has been applied for two reasons. First, I hope to reduce confusion by recognizing complexity. Second, I wish to consider how each phenomenon fits into answers to the two questions raised at the outset.

It would simplify matters if empathy referred to a single object and if everyone agreed on what that object was. Unfortunately, as with many psychological terms, this is not the case. Both *empathy* and *sympathy* (the term with which empathy is most often contrasted) have been used in a variety of ways. Indeed, with remarkable consistency exactly the same state that some scholars have labeled empathy others have labeled sympathy. I have discerned no clear basis—either historical or logical—for favoring one labeling scheme over another. The best one can do is recognize the different phenomena, make clear the labeling scheme one is adopting, and use that scheme consistently.

Not all eight empathy phenomena are relevant to each of the two empathy-related questions. It is worth considering the relation of each phenomenon to each question in turn.

Question 1: How Do We Know Another's Thoughts and Feelings?

Knowing another person's internal state (concept 1) is the phenomenon for which the first question seeks an explanation. Five of the other phenomena have been offered as explanations. Adopting the posture or matching the neural responses of an observed other (concept

2), coming to feel as another person feels (concept 3), intuiting or projecting oneself into another's situation (concept 4), imagining how another is thinking and feeling (concept 5), and imagining how one would think and feel in the other's place (concept 6) have all been invoked to account for our knowledge of another person's thoughts and feelings.

Some accounts focus on only one of these phenomena. For example, a *theory theory* proponent might argue that we can successfully imagine another's internal state (concept 5) by drawing on our lay theories of what people in general, or people with the other's specific characteristics, are likely to think and feel. Other accounts combine several phenomena. A *simulation theory* proponent might argue that by intuiting and projecting oneself into the other's situation (concept 4) or by imagining how one would think and feel in the other's place (concept 6), one comes to feel as the other feels (concept 3), and knowledge of one's own feelings then enables one to know—or to believe one knows—how the other feels (concept 1). Alternatively, one might propose that by automatically adopting the posture or matching the neural responses of the other (concept 2), one comes to feel as the other feels (concept 3), which enables one to know how the other feels (concept 1).

The last two phenomena identified—feeling vicarious personal distress at witnessing another person's suffering (concept 7) and feeling for another who is suffering (concept 8)—are not sources of knowledge (or belief) about another's state; they are reactions to this knowledge. Thus, they are not likely to be invoked to explain how one knows what another is thinking and feeling. Instead, they figure prominently in answers to the second question.

Question 2: What Leads One Person to Respond with Sensitivity and Care to the Suffering of Another?

There is considerable evidence that feeling distress at witnessing another person in distress (concept 7) can produce motivation to help that person. This motivation does not, however, appear to be directed toward the ultimate goal of relieving the other's distress (i.e., altruistic motivation); the motivation appears to be directed toward the ultimate goal of relieving one's own distress (i.e., egoistic motivation; Batson, 1991). As a result, this distress may not lead one to respond with sensitivity to the suffering of another, especially if there is an opportunity to relieve one's own distress without having to relieve the other's distress. The importance of this motivational distinction is underscored by evidence that parents at high risk of abusing a child are the ones who more frequently report distress at seeing an infant cry (concept 7); those at low risk report increased other-oriented feelings—sympathy and compassion (concept 8)—rather than increased distress (Milner, Halsey, & Fultz, 1995).

Feeling for another person who is suffering (concept 8) is the form of empathy most often invoked to explain what leads one person to respond with sensitive care to the suffering of another. This feeling has, in turn, often been related to one or more of the other seven concepts as possible antecedents.

To feel for another, one must think one knows the other's internal state (concept 1) because feeling *for* is based on a perception of the other's welfare (e.g., that your friend is hurt and afraid). To feel for someone does not, however, require that this perception be accurate. It does not even require that this perception match the other's perception of his or her internal state, which is often the standard used in research to define empathic accuracy (e.g., Ickes, 1993). (In this research, the possibility that the other's perception of his or her internal state could be mistaken tends to be ignored. Is it really true, for example, that your friend is not angry?) Of course, action prompted by other-oriented feelings based on erroneous beliefs about the other's state is apt to be misguided, failing to reach the goal of providing sensitive care.

Matching neural representations or mimicking another's posture (concept 2) may facilitate understanding of, or belief about, another's state (concept 1) and thereby induce other-oriented feelings (concept 8). Still, it seems unlikely that either matching or mimicking is necessary or sufficient to produce such feelings. Your friend's tears may have caused you to cry too. But matching her neural state or mimicking her crying was probably not necessary for you to feel sorry for her. More likely, it was the reverse. Her tears made it clear to you how upset she was, and you cried because you felt sorry for her.

Coming to feel as the other feels (concept 3) may also be an important stepping-stone to understanding the other's state (concept 1) and thereby to other-oriented feelings (concept 8). Once again, however, research suggests that it is neither a necessary nor a sufficient precondition (Batson, Early, & Salvarani, 1997). To feel sorry for your friend you need not feel hurt and afraid too. It is enough to know that she is hurt and afraid (concept 1).

Feeling as the other feels may actually inhibit other-oriented feelings if it leads us to become focused on our own emotional state. Sensing the nervousness of other passengers on an airplane in rough weather, I too may become nervous. If I focus on my own nervousness, not theirs, I am likely to feel less for them, not more.

Intuiting or projecting oneself into another's situation (concept 4) may give one a lively sense of what the other is thinking and feeling (concept 1) and may thereby facilitate other-oriented feelings (concept 8). But when the state of the other is obvious because of what has happened or been said, intuition or projection is probably unnecessary. And when the other's state is not obvious, intuition or projection runs the risk of imposing an interpretation of the other's state that is inaccurate, especially if one does not have a precise understanding of relevant differences between oneself and the other.

Instructions to imagine how the other is feeling (concept 5) have often been used to induce other-oriented feelings for a person in need (concept 8) in participants in laboratory experiments (see Batson, 1991, for a review). Still, this imagine-other perspective should not be confused or equated with the other-oriented emotion it evokes (Coke, Batson, & McDavis, 1978).

When attending to another person in distress, imagining how you would think and feel in that situation (concept 6) may stimulate other-oriented feelings (concept 8). However, this imagine-self perspective is also likely to elicit self-oriented feelings of distress (concept 7; see Batson, Early, & Salvarani, 1997; Stotland, 1969). If the other's situation is unfamiliar or unclear, then imagining how you would think and feel in that situation may provide a useful, possibly essential, basis for perceiving the other's state (concept 1), a necessary precondition for experiencing other-oriented feelings. But once again, if the other differs from you, then focusing on how you would think and feel may prove misleading. And if the other's situation is familiar or clear, then to imagine how you would think and feel in that situation may actually inhibit other-oriented feelings (Nickerson, 1999). As you listened to your friend talk about losing her job, your thoughts about how you would feel if you lost your own job led you to become self-concerned, to feel anxious and uneasy—and lucky by comparison. These reactions likely dampened your other-oriented feelings of sorrow for her.

Because of prominence and popularity, I have dwelt on other-oriented feelings (concept 8) as a source of sensitive response to the suffering of others. But several of the other phenomena called empathy have been offered as sources of sensitive response, independent of mediation through other-oriented feelings for the sufferer. For example, it has been suggested that coming to feel as another person feels (concept 3)—perhaps combined with an imagine-other perspective (concept 5)—can lead us to respond directly to the other's suffering as we would to our own (Preston & de Waal, 2002). It has also been suggested that imagining how one would think and feel in the other's place (concept 6) can lead directly to a more sensitive response to the plight of members of stereotyped out-groups (Galinsky & Moskowitz, 2000).

For those whose profession commits them to helping others in need (such as clinicians, counselors, and physicians), accurate perception of the need—diagnosis—is of paramount importance because one is not likely to address a need effectively unless one recognizes it. Moreover, high emotional arousal, including arousal of other-oriented emotions, may interfere with one's ability to help effectively (MacLean, 1967). Accordingly, within the helping professions, emphasis is often placed on accurate knowledge of the client's or patient's internal state (concept 1), not on other-oriented feelings (concept 8), as the key source of effective response to need.

Conclusion

Distinctions among the various things called empathy are sometimes subtle, yet there seems little doubt that each exists. Most are familiar experiences. Their familiarity should not, however, lead us to ignore their significance. The processes whereby one person can come to know the internal state of another and can be motivated to respond with sensitive care are of enormous importance for our life together. Some great thinkers, such as the philosopher David Hume, have suggested that these processes are the basis for all social perception and interaction. They are certainly key elements of our social nature.

To recognize the distinctiveness of these eight things called empathy complicates matters. Still, it seems essential if we are to understand these phenomena and how they relate to one another. It also seems essential if we are to advance our understanding of how it is possible to know the internal states of others and to respond with sensitivity to their suffering. Fortunately, social neuroscience has already begun to recognize at least some of the distinctions, and has begun to identify their neural substrates (see, for example, Jackson, et al., 2006; Lamm, Batson, & Decety, 2007; Singer et al., 2004).

Acknowledgments

Thanks to Nadia Ahmad, Tobias Gschwendner, Jakob Eklund, Luis Oceja, Adam Powell, and Eric Stocks for helpful comments on a draft.

Note

1. I am certainly not the first to note a range of empathy-related concepts (see Becker, 1931; Reik, 1948; Scheler, 1913/1970). But as the intellectual landscape has changed, the relevant conceptual distinctions have also changed. Therefore, I shall not present earlier attempts at conceptual clarification.

References

Adolphs, R. (1999). Social cognition and the human brain. *Trends in Cognitive Sciences*, *3*, 469–479.

Barrett-Lennard, G. T. (1981). The empathy cycle: Refinement of a nuclear concept. *Journal of Counseling Psychology*, *28*, 91–100.

Batson, C. D. (1991). *The altruism question: Toward a social-psychological answer*. Hillsdale, NJ: Erlbaum.

Batson, C. D., Early, S., & Salvarani, G. (1997). Perspective taking: Imagining how another feels versus imagining how you would feel. *Personality and Social Psychology Bulletin*, *23*, 751–758.

Bavelas, J. B., Black, A., Lemery, C. R., & Mullett, J. (1986). "I show you how you feel": Motor mimicry as a communicative act. *Journal of Personality and Social Psychology*, *50*, 322–329.

Becker, H. (1931). Some forms of sympathy: A phenomenological analysis. *Journal of Abnormal and Social Psychology*, *26*, 58–68.

Coke, J. S., Batson, C. D., & McDavis, K. (1978). Empathic mediation of helping: A two-stage model. *Journal of Personality and Social Psychology*, *36*, 752–766.

Damasio, A. R. (2003). *Looking for Spinoza: Joy, sorrow, and the feeling brain*. Orlando, FL: Harcourt.

Darwall, S. (1998). Empathy, sympathy, care. *Philosophical Studies*, *89*, 261–282.

Decety, J., & Chaminade, T. (2003). Neural correlates of feeling sympathy. *Neuropsychologia, 41*, 127–138.

Dimberg, U., Thunberg, M., & Elmehed, K. (2000). Unconscious facial reactions to emotional facial expressions. *Psychological Science, 11*, 86–89.

Eisenberg, N., & Strayer, J. (Eds.). (1987). *Empathy and its development.* New York: Cambridge University Press.

Eslinger, P. J. (1998). Neurological and neuropsychological bases of empathy. *European Neurology, 1998*, 193–199.

Galinsky, A. D., & Moskowitz, G. B. (2000). Perspective-taking: Decreasing stereotype expression, stereotype accessibility, and in-group favoritism. *Journal of Personality and Social Psychology, 78*, 708–724.

Gordon, R. M. (1995). Sympathy, simulation, and the impartial spectator. *Ethics, 105*, 727–742.

Hatfield, E., Cacioppo, J. T., & Rapson, R. L. (1994). *Emotional contagion.* New York: Cambridge University Press.

Hodges, S. D., & Wegner, D. M. (1997). Automatic and controlled empathy. In W. Ickes (Ed.), *Empathic accuracy* (pp. 311–339). New York: Guilford Press.

Hoffman, M. L. (1981). The development of empathy. In J. P. Rushton & R. M. Sorrentino (Eds.), *Altruism and helping behavior: Social, personality, and developmental perspectives* (pp. 41–63). Hillsdale, NJ: Erlbaum.

Hoffman, M. L. (2000). *Empathy and moral development: Implications for caring and justice.* New York: Cambridge University Press.

Hume, D. (1740/1896). *A treatise of human nature* (L. A. Selby-Bigge, Ed.). Oxford: Oxford University Press.

Ickes, W. (1993). Empathic accuracy. *Journal of Personality, 61*, 587–610.

Jackson, P. L., Brunet, E., Meltzoff, A. N., & Decety, J. (2006). Empathy examined through the neural mechanisms involved in imagining how I feel versus how you feel pain. *Neuropsychologia, 44*, 752–761.

Krebs, D. L. (1975). Empathy and altruism. *Journal of Personality and Social Psychology, 32*, 1134–1146.

LaFrance, M., & Ickes, W. (1981). Posture mirroring and interactional involvement: Sex and sex typing influences. *Journal of Nonverbal Behavior, 5*, 139–154.

Lamm, C., Batson, C. D., & Decety, J. (2007). The neural substrate of human empathy: Effects of perspective-taking and cognitive appraisal. *Journal of Cognitive Neuroscience, 19*, 1–17.

Levenson, R. W., & Ruef, A. M. (1992). Empathy: A physiological substrate. *Journal of Personality and Social Psychology, 63*, 234–246.

Lipps, T. (1903). Einfühlung, inner Nachahmung, und Organ-empfindungen. *Archiv für die gesamte Psychologie, 1*, 185–204.

MacLean, P. D. (1967). The brain in relation to empathy and medical education. *Journal of Nervous and Mental Disease, 144*, 374–382.

Mead, G. H. (1934). *Mind, self, and society*. Chicago: University of Chicago Press.

Meltzoff, A. N., & Moore, M. K. (1997). Explaining facial imitation: A theoretical model. *Early Development and Parenting, 6*, 179–192.

Milner, J. S., Halsey, L. B., & Fultz, J. (1995). Empathic responsiveness and affective reactivity to infant stimuli in high- and low-risk for physical child abuse mothers. *Child Abuse and Neglect, 19*, 767–780.

Nickerson, R. S. (1999). How we know—and sometimes misjudge—what others know: Imputing one's own knowledge to others. *Psychological Bulletin, 125*, 737–759.

Piaget, J. (1953). *The origins of intelligence in the child*. New York: International Universities Press.

Povinelli, D. J. (1993). Reconstructing the evolution of mind. *American Psychologist, 48*, 493–509.

Preston, S. D., & de Waal, F. B. M. (2002). Empathy: Its ultimate and proximate bases. *Behavioral and Brain Sciences, 25*, 1–72.

Reik, T. (1948). *Listening with the third ear: The inner experience of a psychoanalyst*. New York: Farrar, Straus.

Ruby, P., & Decety, J. (2004). How would you feel versus how do you think she would feel? A neuroimaging study of perspective taking with social emotions. *Journal of Cognitive Neuroscience, 16*, 988–999.

Sagi, A., & Hoffman, M. L. (1976). Empathic distress in the newborn. *Developmental Psychology, 12*, 175–176.

Scheler, M. (1913/1970). *The nature of sympathy* (P. Heath, Trans.). Hamden, CT: Archon Books.

Singer, T., Seymour, B., O'Doherty, J., Kaube, H., Dolan, R. J., & Frith, C. D. (2004). Empathy for pain involves the affective but not sensory components of pain. *Science, 303*, 1157–1162.

Smith, A. (1759/1853). *The theory of moral sentiments*. London: Alex Murray.

Sober, E., & Wilson, D. S. (1998). *Unto others: The evolution and psychology of unselfish behavior*. Cambridge, MA: Harvard University Press.

Stotland, E. (1969). Exploratory investigations of empathy. In L. Berkowitz (Ed.), *Advances in experimental social psychology* (Vol. 4, pp. 271–313). New York: Academic Press.

Titchener, E. B. (1909). *Lectures on the experimental psychology of the thought processes*. New York: Macmillan.

Tomasello, M. (1999). *The cultural origins of human cognition*. Cambridge, MA: Harvard University Press.

Wispé, L. (1968). Sympathy and empathy. In D. L. Sills (Ed.), *International encyclopedia of the social sciences* (Vol. 15, pp. 441–447). New York: Free Press.

Wispé, L. (1986). The distinction between sympathy and empathy: To call forth a concept a word is needed. *Journal of Personality and Social Psychology, 50,* 314–321.

Zahn-Waxler, C., Robinson, J. L., & Emde, R. N. (1992). The development of empathy in twins. *Developmental Psychology, 28,* 1038–1047.

II Social, Cognitive, and Developmental Perspectives on Empathy

2   Emotional Contagion and Empathy

Elaine Hatfield, Richard L. Rapson, and Yen-Chi L. Le

Whoever battles with monsters had better see that it does not turn him into a monster. And if you gaze long into an abyss, the abyss will gaze back into you.
—Nietzsche

Today there are many definitions of empathy. Most clinical and counseling psychologists, however, agree that true empathy requires three distinct skills: the ability to share the other person's feelings, the cognitive ability to intuit what another person is feeling, and a "socially beneficial" intention to respond compassionately to that person's distress (Decety & Jackson, 2004). This chapter focuses on the second of these processes: the ability of people to "feel themselves into" another's emotions via the process of emotional contagion. We review what is known about this pervasive phenomenon, discuss three mechanisms that may account for it, and propose questions for further research.

Scholars from a variety of disciplines—neuroscience, biology, social psychology, sociology, and life-span psychology—have proposed that *primitive emotional contagion* is of critical importance in understanding human cognition, emotion, and behavior. Primitive emotional contagion is a basic building block of human interaction, assisting in "mind reading" and allowing people to understand and to share the feelings of others.

Emotional contagion is best conceptualized as a multiply determined family of social, psychophysiological, and behavioral phenomena. Theorists disagree as to what constitutes an emotion family. Most, however, would agree that emotional "packages" comprise many components—including conscious awareness; facial, vocal, and postural expression; neurophysiological and autonomic nervous system activity; and instrumental behaviors. Different portions of the brain may process the various aspects of emotion. However, because the brain integrates the emotional information it receives, each of the emotional components acts on and is acted upon by the others (see Hatfield, Cacioppo, & Rapson, 1994, for a discussion of this point).

Hatfield, Cacioppo, and Rapson (1994) define primitive *emotional contagion* as "the tendency to automatically mimic and synchronize facial expressions, vocalizations, postures, and movements with those of another person and, consequently, to converge emotionally" (p. 5).

The Emotional Contagion Scale was designed to assess people's susceptibility to "catching" joy and happiness, love, fear and anxiety, anger, and sadness and depression, as well as emotions in general (see Doherty, 1997; Hatfield, Cacioppo, & Rapson, 1994). The Emotional Contagion Scale has been translated into a variety of languages, including Finnish, German, Greek, Indian (Hindi), Japanese, Portuguese, and Swedish. (For information on the reliability and validity of this scale, see Doherty, 1997).

Possible Mechanisms of Emotional Contagion

Theoretically, emotions can be caught in several ways. Early investigators proposed that conscious reasoning, analysis, and imagination accounted for the phenomenon. For example, the economic philosopher Adam Smith (1759/1966) observed:

> Though our brother is upon the rack . . . by the imagination we place ourselves in his situation, we conceive ourselves enduring all the same torments, we enter as it were into his body, and become in some measure the same person with him, and thence form some idea of his sensations, and even feel something which, though weaker in degree, is not altogether unlike them. (p. 9)

However, primitive emotional contagion appears to be a far more subtle, automatic, and ubiquitous process than theorists such as Smith supposed. There is considerable evidence, for instance, in support of the following propositions:

Proposition 1: Mimicry

In conversation, people automatically and continuously mimic and synchronize their movements with the facial expressions, voices, postures, movements, and instrumental behaviors of others.

Scientists and writers have long observed that people tend to mimic the emotional expressions of others. As early as 1759, Adam Smith (1759/1966) acknowledged that as people imagine themselves in another's situation, they display motor mimicry: "When we see a stroke aimed, and just ready to fall upon the leg or arm of another person, we naturally shrink and draw back on our leg or our own arm" (p. 4).

Smith felt that such imitation was "almost a reflex." Later, Theodor Lipps (1903) suggested that conscious empathy is attributable to the instinctive motor mimicry of another person's expressions of affect. Since the 1700s, researchers have collected considerable evidence that people do tend to imitate others' emotional expressions.

Facial Mimicry   The fact that people's faces often mirror the facial expressions of those around them is well documented (Dimberg, 1982; Vaughan & Lanzetta, 1980). Neuroscientists and social-psychophysiologists, for example, have found that people's cognitive responses (as measured by functional magnetic resonance imaging [fMRI] techniques) and facial expressions (as measured by electromyography [EMG]) tend to reflect the most subtle of moment-to-moment changes in the emotional expressions of those they observe (Wild et al., 2003). This motor mimicry is often so swift and so subtle that it produces no observable change in facial expression (Lundqvist, 1995).

Lars-Olov Lundqvist (1995) recorded Swedish college students' facial EMG activity as they studied photographs of target persons who displayed happy, sad, angry, fearful, surprised, and disgusted facial expressions. He found that the various target faces evoked very different EMG response patterns. When participants observed happy facial expressions, they showed increased muscular activity over the *zygomaticus major* (cheek) muscle region. When they observed angry facial expressions, they displayed increased muscular activity over the *corrugator supercilii* (brow) muscle region.

A great deal of research has documented the fact that infants (Meltzoff & Prinz, 2002), young children, adolescents, and adults automatically mimic other people's facial expressions of emotion (see Hatfield, Cacioppo, & Rapson, 1994; Hurley & Chater, 2005b, for a review of this research). For a review of the factors that shape the likelihood that people will or will not mimic others' emotional expressions, see Hess & Blair, 2001; Hess & Bourgeois, 2006).

Vocal Mimicry People have also been shown to mimic and synchronize vocal utterances. Different people prefer different interaction tempos. When partners interact, if things are to go well, their speech cycles must become mutually entrained. There is a good deal of evidence from research using controlled interview settings that supports interspeaker influence in speech rates, utterance durations, and latencies of response (see Cappella & Planalp, 1981; Chapple, 1982).

Postural Mimicry Individuals have also been found to mimic and synchronize their postures and movements (Bernieri, et al., 1991; see Hatfield, Cacioppo, & Rapson, 1994, for a summary of this research).

We are probably not able *consciously* to mimic others very effectively; the process is simply too complex and too fast. For example, it took even the lightning-fast Muhammad Ali a minimum of 190 milliseconds to detect a signal light and 40 milliseconds more to throw a punch in response. Yet, William Condon and W. D. Ogston (1966) found that college students could synchronize their movements within 21 milliseconds (the time of one picture frame). Mark Davis (1985) argues that microsynchrony is mediated by brain structures at multiple levels of the neuraxis and is either "something you've got or something you don't"; there is no way that one can deliberately 'do' it" (p. 69). Those who try consciously to mirror others, he speculates, are doomed to look "phony."

In sum, there is considerable evidence that people are capable of automatically mimicking and synchronizing their faces, vocal productions, postures, and movements with those around them. They do this with startling rapidity, automatically mimicking and synchronizing a surprising number of emotional characteristics in a single instant (Condon, 1982).

Proposition 2: Feedback

Proposition 2: People's emotional experience is affected, moment to moment, by the activation of and/or feedback from facial, vocal, postural, and movement mimicry.

Theoretically, participants' emotional experience could be influenced by (1) the central nervous system commands that direct such mimicry/synchrony in the first place; (2) the afferent feedback from such facial, verbal, or postural mimicry/synchrony; or (3) conscious self-perception processes, wherein individuals make inferences about their own emotional states on the basis of their own expressive behavior. Given the functional redundancy that exists across levels of the neuraxis, all three processes may operate to insure that emotional experience is shaped by facial, vocal, and postural mimicry/synchrony and expression.

Recent reviews of the literature tend to agree that emotions are tempered to some extent by facial, vocal, and postural feedback.

Facial Feedback Darwin (1872/2005) argued that emotional experience should be profoundly affected by feedback from the facial muscles:

The free expression by outward signs of an emotion intensifies it. On the other hand, the repression, as far as is possible of all outward signs, softens our emotions. He who gives way to violent gestures will increase rage; he who does not control the signs of fear will experience fear in a greater degree; and he who remains passive when overwhelmed with grief loses his best chance of recovering elasticity of mind. (p. 365)

Researchers have tested the facial feedback hypothesis, using a variety of strategies to induce participants to adopt emotional facial expressions. Sometimes experimenters simply ask participants to exaggerate or to try to hide any emotional reactions they might have. Second, they sometimes try to "trick" participants into adopting various facial expressions. Third, they sometimes arrange things so that participants will unconsciously mimic the emotional facial expressions of others. In all three types of experiments, people's emotional experiences tend to be affected by the facial expressions they adopt (Adelmann & Zajonc, 1989; Matsumoto, 1987.)

In a classic experiment, James Laird and Charles Bresler (1992) told participants that they were interested in studying the action of facial muscles. Their experimental room contained apparatus designed to convince anyone that complicated multichannel recordings were about to be made of facial muscle activity. Silver cup electrodes were attached to the participants' faces between their eyebrows, at the corners of their mouths, and at the corners of their jaws. The electrodes were connected via an impressive tangle of strings and wires to electronic apparatus (which in fact served no function at all.) The experimenter then proceeded surreptitiously to arrange the faces of the participants into emotional expressions. The authors found that emotional attributions *were* shaped, in part, by changes in the facial musculature. Participants in the "frown" condition reported being less happy (and more angry) than those in the "smile" condition. The participants' comments give us some idea of how this process worked. One man said with a kind of puzzlement:

> When my jaw was clenched and my brows down, I tried not to be angry but it just fit the position. I'm not in any angry mood but I found my thoughts wandering to things that made me angry, which is sort of silly I guess. I knew I was in an experiment and knew I had no reason to feel that way, but I just lost control. (p. 480)

Paul Ekman and his colleagues have argued that both emotional experience *and* autonomic nervous system (ANS) activity are affected by facial feedback (Ekman, Levenson, & Friesen, 1983). They asked people to produce six emotions: surprise, disgust, sadness, anger, fear, and happiness. They were to do this either by reliving times when they had experienced such emotions or by arranging their facial muscles in appropriate poses. The authors found that the act of reliving emotional experiences or flexing facial muscles into characteristic emotional expressions produced effects on the ANS that would normally accompany such emotions. Thus, facial expressions seemed to be capable of generating appropriate ANS arousal.

Vocal Feedback   An array of evidence supports the contention that subjective emotional experience is affected, moment to moment, by the activation of and/or feedback from vocal mimicry (Duclos et al., 1989; Hatfield, Cacioppo, & Rapson, 1994; Hatfield et al., 1995; Zajonc, Murphy, & Inglehart, 1989).

Elaine Hatfield and her colleagues (1995) conducted a series of experiments designed to test the vocal feedback hypothesis. Participants were men and women of African, Chinese, European, Filipino, Hawaiian, Hispanic, Japanese, Korean, Pacific Island, or mixed ancestry. The authors made every effort to hide the fact that they were interested in the participants' emotions. (They claimed that Bell Telephone was testing the ability of various kinds of telephone systems to reproduce the human voice faithfully.) Participants were then led to private rooms, where the experimenter gave them a cassette tape containing one of six sound patterns, one a neutral control and the others corresponding to joy, love/tenderness, sadness, fear, and anger.

Communication researchers have documented that the basic emotions are linked with specific patterns of intonation, vocal quality, rhythm, and pausing. When people are happy, for example, they produce sounds with small amplitude variation, large pitch variation, fast tempo, a sharp sound envelope, and few harmonics. In the study by Hatfield and her colleagues, the first five tapes were therefore designed to exhibit the sound patterns appropriate to their respective emotions. Specifically, the joyous sounds had some of the qualities of merry laughter; the sad sounds possessed the qualities of crying; the companionate love tape consisted of a series of soft "ooohs" and "aaahs"; the angry tape comprised a series of low growling noises from the throat; and the fearful sounds included a set of short, sharp cries and gasps. Finally, the neutral tape was one long monotone, a hum, without any breaks. Participants were asked to reproduce the sounds as exactly as possible into a telephone. Results revealed that participants' emotions were powerfully affected in the predicted ways by the specific sounds they produced. This experiment therefore provided additional support for the vocal feedback hypothesis.

Postural Feedback   Finally, there is evidence suggesting that emotions are shaped by feedback from posture and movement (see Bernieri, Reznick, & Rosenthal, 1988; Duclos et al., 1989; and Hatfield, Cacioppo, & Rapson, 1994, for a review of this research). Interestingly, the theorist of theater Konstantin Stanislavski noticed the connection between posture and performance (Moore, 1984). He argued, "Emotional memory stores our past experiences; to relive them, actors must execute indispensable, logical physical actions in the given circumstances. There are as many nuances of emotions as there are physical actions" (pp. 52–53).

Stanislavski proposed that we may relive emotions any time we engage in a variety of small actions that were once associated with those emotions.

In a variety of studies, then, we find evidence that people tend to feel emotions consistent with the facial, vocal, and postural expressions they adopt. The link between facial, vocal, and postural expression appears to be very specific: when people produce expressions of fear, anger, sadness, or disgust, they are more likely to feel not just any unpleasant emotion, but the emotion associated with those *specific* expressions; for example, those who make a sad expression feel sad, not angry (see Duclos et al., 1989). What remains unclear is how important such feedback is (is it necessary, sufficient, or merely a small part of emotional experience?) and exactly how the physical expression and the emotion are linked (see Adelmann & Zajonc, 1989). (For a critical review of this literature see Manstead, 1988).

Proposition 3: Contagion

As a consequence of mimicry and feedback, people tend, from moment to moment, to "catch" others' emotions.

Researchers from a variety of disciplines have provided evidence in support of this contention. Recently, discoveries in neuroscience have provided some insight into *why* people so readily "catch" the emotions of others and why it is so easy to empathize with other people's thoughts, emotions, and behaviors. Some examples follow.

Neuroscientists contend that certain neurons (canonical neurons) provide a direct link between perception and action. Other types of neurons (mirror neurons) fire when a certain type of action is performed *and* when primates observe another animal performing the same kind of action. Scientists propose that such brain circuits might account for emotional contagion and empathy in primates, including humans (see Iacoboni, 2005; Rizzolatti, 2005; Wild, Erb, & Bartels, 2001; Wild et al., 2003).

The real question, of course, is, What is the sequential order of mirror neuron firing and mimicry? Iacoboni and his colleagues contend that their monkeys are "doing nothing"—simply observing the other animal—when the mirror-neuron firing occurs (see Iacoboni, 2005; Rizzolatti, 2005; Wild et al., 2001, 2003). We know that this is not so. At every instant, the primate is mimicking the stimulus person's (or monkey's) face, voice, and posture. Depending on the timing, the mirror-neuron firing may *cause* the monkey's mimicked grasping, or the animal's mimicked grasping may cause the firing in the location under study. That is, the same brain areas may fire when an animal intentionally acts and when it performs the same action via mimicry. Only subsequent research will tell. Both processes, of course, would be of great interest to emotional contagion researchers.

Blakemore and Frith (2005) have argued that imagining, observing, or in any way preparing to perform an action excites the same motor programs used to execute that same action. They review a great deal of recent research demonstrating that, in humans, several brain regions (specifically the premotor and parietal cortices) are activated both during action generation and during the observation of others' actions. The premotor resonance was not dependent on the motive having a goal, whereas the parietal cortex was activated only when the action was directed toward a goal. Some have argued that this mirror system allows us to plan our own actions and also to understand the actions of others.

In the 1950s, primatologists conducted a great deal of research indicating that animals do seem to catch others' emotions. R. E. Miller and his colleagues (Miller, Banks, & Ogawa, 1963), for example, found that monkeys often transmit their fears to their peers. The faces, voices, and postures of frightened monkeys serve as warnings; they signal potential trouble. Monkeys catch the fear of others and thus are primed to make appropriate avoidance responses. Ethologists argue that the imitation of emotional expression constitutes a phylogenetically ancient and basic form of intraspecies communication. Such contagion also appears in many vertebrate species, including mice (Brothers, 1989; Mogil, 2006).

Scholars from a variety of disciplines provide evidence that people do in fact catch one another's emotions: there is evidence from clinical observers (Coyne, 1976), social psychologists and sociologists (Hatfield, Cacioppo, & Rapson, 1994; Le Bon, 1896; Tseng & Hsu, 1980), neuroscientists and primatologists (Hurley & Chater, 2005a; Wild et al., 2003), life span researchers (Hurley & Chater, 2005a, 2005b), and historians (Klawans, 1990) suggesting that people may indeed catch the emotions of others at all times, in all societies, and perhaps on very large scales. (See Hatfield, Cacioppo, & Rapson, 1994; Wild, Erb, & Bartels, 2001; Wild et al., 2003, for a summary of this research.)

Summary

In theory, the process of emotional contagion consists of three stages: mimicry, feedback, and contagion. People tend (a) to automatically mimic the facial expressions, vocal expressions, postures, and instrumental behaviors of those around them, and thereby (b) to feel a pale reflection of others' emotions as a consequence of such feedback. The result is that people tend (c) to catch one another's emotions. Presumably, when people automatically mimic their companions' fleeting facial, vocal, and postural expressions of emotion, they often come to feel a pale reflection of their companions' actual emotions. By attending to this stream of tiny moment-to-moment reactions, people are able to "feel themselves into" the emotional lives of others. They can track the intentions and feelings of others moment to moment, even when they are not explicitly attending to the information.

Implications of Existing Research

In this chapter we confront a paradox. People seem to be capable of mimicking others' facial, vocal, and postural expressions with stunning rapidity. As a consequence, they are able to feel themselves into those other emotional lives to a surprising extent. And yet, puzzlingly, most people seem oblivious to the importance of mimicry and synchrony in social encounters. They seem unaware of how swiftly and how completely they are able to track the expressive behaviors and emotions of others.

What are some implications of recent findings concerning the nature of contagion and empathy? The research on contagion underscores the fact that we use multiple means to gain information about others' emotional states: Conscious analytic skills can certainly help us figure out what makes people "tick." But if we pay careful attention to the emotions we experience in the company of others, we may well gain an extra edge by feeling ourselves into the emotional states of others. In fact, there is evidence that both what we *think* and what we *feel* may provide valuable, but different, information about others. In one study, for example, Christopher Hsee and his colleagues found that people's conscious assessments of what others "must be" feeling were heavily influenced by what those others *said*. People's own emotions, however, were more influenced by the others' nonverbal clues as to what they were really feeling (Hsee, Hatfield, & Chemtob, 1992).

Proposed Questions

In recent years, emotional contagion has been cited to explain the thoughts, feelings, and behavior of people in general, and, more specifically of children with autism (Decety & Jackson, 2004; Hurley & Chater, 2005a, 2005b; music lovers (Davies, 2006), religious fanatics, terrorists, and suicide bombers (Hatfield & Rapson, 2004), people who die by suicide, and people in crowds (Adamatzky, 2005; Fischer, 1995), to name just a few. What scientists haven't yet done is explore some of the basic questions concerning who is susceptible to (or resistant to) emotional contagion and under what conditions.

A number of important questions remain to be answered as investigators seek to understand this important component of empathy, primitive emotional contagion.

1. What kinds of *people* are most vulnerable to catching others' emotions?
2. In what kinds of *relationships* are people most vulnerable to contagion?
3. What are the advantages (or disadvantages) of possessing the power to "infect" others with one's own emotions? What are the advantages (disadvantages) of possessing the sensitivity to read and reflect others' emotions?
4. Are people better liked when they possess a natural tendency to mimic others' emotional expressions and behaviors? What happens when people consciously try to imitate others' emotional expressions and behaviors? Does that make people like them more or less, since their performance will always be a little bit "off"?
5. Can people be taught to be more in tune with others' emotions (i.e., to be more susceptible to emotional contagion?)
6. Can people be taught to resist being overwhelmed by others' emotions (i.e., to become less susceptible to emotional contagion?)

The answers to these questions await the attention of researchers, for many of whom the study of emotional contagion has acquired its own contagious appeal.

References

Adamatzky, A. (2005). *Dynamics of Crowd-Minds: Patterns of irrationality in emotions, beliefs and actions.* London: World Scientific.

Adelmann, P. K., & Zajonc, R. B. (1989). Facial efference and the experience of emotion. *Annual Review of Psychology, 40,* 249–280.

Bernieri, F. J., Davis, J. M., Knee, C. R., & Rosenthal, R. (1991). *Interactional synchrony and the social affordance of rapport: A validation study.* Unpublished manuscript, Oregon State University, Corvallis.

Bernieri, F. J., Reznick, J. S., & Rosenthal, R. (1988). Synchrony, pseudosynchrony, and dissynchrony: Measuring the entrainment process in mother–infant interactions. *Journal of Personality and Social Psychology, 54,* 243–253.

Blakemore, S. J., & Frith, C. D. (2005). The role of motor cognition in the prediction of action. *Neuropsychologia, 43 (2),* 260–267.

Brothers, L. (1989). A biological perspective on empathy. *American Journal of Psychiatry, 146,* 10–19.

Cappella, J. N., & Planalp, S. (1981). Talk and silence sequences in informal conversations: III. Interspeaker influence. *Human Communication Research, 7,* 117–132.

Chapple, E. D. (1982). Movement and sound: The musical language of body rhythms in interaction. In M. Davis (Ed.), *Interaction rhythms: Periodicity in communicative behavior* (pp. 31–52). New York: Human Sciences Press.

Condon, W. S. (1982). Cultural microrhythms. In M. Davis (Ed.), *Interaction rhythms: Periodicity in communicative behavior* (pp. 53–76). New York: Human Sciences Press.

Condon, W. S., & Ogston, W. D. (1966). Sound film analysis of normal and pathological behavior patterns. *Journal of Nervous and Mental Disease, 143*, 338–347.

Coyne, J. C. (1976). Depression and the response of others. *Journal of Abnormal Psychology, 85*, 186–193.

Darwin, C. (1872/2005). *The expression of the emotions in man and animals.* Whitefish, MT: Kessinger Publishing.

Davies, S. (2006). Infectious music: Music-listener emotional contagion. Paper presented at the Conference on Empathy, California State University, Fullerton.

Davis, M. R. (1985). Perceptual and affective reverberation components. In A. B. Goldstein & G. Y. Michaels (Eds.), *Empathy: Development, training, and consequences* (pp. 62–108). Hillsdale, NJ: Erlbaum.

Decety, J., & Jackson, P. L. (2004). The functional architecture of human empathy. *Behavioral and Cognitive Neuroscience Reviews, 3*, 71–100.

Dimberg, U. (1982). Facial reactions to facial expressions. *Psychophysiology, 19*, 643–647.

Doherty, R. W. (1997). The Emotional Contagion scale: A measure of individual differences. *Journal of Nonverbal Behavior, 21*, 131–154.

Duclos, S. E., Laird, J. D., Schneider, E., Sexter, M., Stern, L., & Van Lighten, O. (1989). Emotion-specific effects of facial expressions and postures on emotional experience. *Journal of Personality and Social Psychology, 57*, 100–108.

Ekman, P., Levenson, R. W., & Friesen, W. V. (1983). Autonomic nervous system activity distinguishes among emotions. *Science, 221*, 1208–1210.

Fischer, A. H. (1995). *Emotional contagion in intergroup contexts.* Netherlands: European Science Foundation, Open MAGW Program, NWO grant 461-04-650.

Hatfield, E., Cacioppo, J., & Rapson, R. L. (1994). *Emotional contagion.* New York: Cambridge University Press.

Hatfield, E., Hsee, C. K., Costello, J., Weisman, M. S., & Denney, C. (1995). The impact of vocal feedback on emotional experience and expression. *Journal of Social Behavior and Personality, 10*, 293–312.

Hatfield, E., & Rapson, R. L. (2004). Emotional contagion: Religious and ethnic hatreds and global terrorism. In L. Z. Tiedens & C. W. Leach (Eds.), *The social life of emotions* (pp. 129–143). Cambridge: Cambridge University Press, pp. 129–143.

Hess, U., and Blair, S. (2001). Facial mimicry and emotional contagion to dynamic emotional facial expressions and their influence on decoding accuracy. *International Journal of Psychophysiology, 40*, 129–141.

Hess, U., & Bourgeois, P. (2006, January 27). *The social costs of mimicking: Why we should not both look angry.* Paper presented at the Society for Personality and Social Psychology, Palm Springs, FL.

Hsee, C. K., Hatfield, E., & Chemtob, C. (1992). Assessments of emotional states of others: Conscious judgments versus emotional contagion. *Journal of Social and Clinical Psychology, 2*, 119–128.

Hurley, S., & Chater, N. (2005a). *Perspectives on imitation: From neuroscience to social science: Vol. 1. Mechanisms of imitation and imitation in animals.* Cambridge, MA: MIT Press.

Hurley, S., & Chater, N. (2005b). *Perspectives on imitation: From neuroscience to social science: Vol. 2. Imitation, human development, and culture.* Cambridge, MA: MIT Press.

Iacoboni, M. (2005). Understanding others: Imitation, language, and empathy. In S. Hurley & N. Chater, *Perspectives on imitation: From neuroscience to social science: Vol. 1. Mechanisms of imitation and imitation in animals* (pp. 77–101). Cambridge, MA: MIT Press.

Klawans, H. L. (1990). *Newton's madness: Further tales of clinical neurology.* London: Headline Book Publishers.

Laird, J. D., & Bresler, C. (1992). The process of emotional feeling: A self-perception theory. Reported in M. Clark (Ed.), *Emotion: Review of Personality and Social Psychology, 13*, 213–234.

Le Bon, G. (1896). *The crowd: A study of the popular mind.* London: Ernest Benn.

Lipps, T. (1903). Kapitel: Die einfühlung. In *Leitfaden der psychologie* [Guide to psychology] (pp. 187–201). Leipzig: Verlag von Wilhelm Engelmann.

Lundqvist, L. O. (1995). Facial EMG reactions to facial expressions: A case of facial emotional contagion? *Scandinavian Journal of Psychology, 36*, 130–141.

Manstead, A. S. R. (1988). The role of facial movement in emotion. In H. L. Wagner (Ed.), *Social psychophysiology and emotion: Theory and clinical applications* (pp. 105–130). New York: Wiley.

Matsumoto, D. (1987). The role of facial response in the experience of emotion: More methodological problems and a meta-analysis. *Journal of Personality and Social Psychology, 52*, 769–774.

Meltzoff, A. M., & Prinz, W. (Eds.). (2002). *The imitative mind: Development, evaluation, and brain bases.* Cambridge: Cambridge University Press.

Miller, R. E., Banks, J. H., & Ogawa, N. (1963). Role of facial expression in "cooperative-avoidance conditioning" in monkeys. *Journal of Abnormal and Social Psychology, 67*, 24–30.

Mogil, J. (2006, July 4). Mice show evidence of empathy. *The Scientist: Magazine of the Life Sciences* http//www.the-scientist.com/news/display/23764. Accessed July 1, 2007.

Moore, S. (1984). *The Stanislavski system.* New York: Viking.

Rizzolatti, G. (2005). The mirror neuron system and imitation. In S. Hurley & N. Chater, *Perspectives on imitation: From neuroscience to social science: Vol. 1. Mechanisms of imitation and imitation in animals* (pp. 55–76). Cambridge, MA: MIT Press.

Smith, A. (1759/1976). *The theory of moral sentiments*. Oxford: Clarendon Press.

Tseng, W-S., & Hsu, J. (1980). Minor psychological disturbances of everyday life. In H. C. Triandis & J. D. Draguns (Eds.), *Handbook of cross-cultural psychology: Vol. 6. Psychopathology* (pp. 61–97). Boston: Allyn & Bacon.

Vaughan, K. B., & Lanzetta, J. T. (1980). Vicarious instigation and conditioning of facial expressive and autonomic responses to a model's expressive display of pain. *Journal of Personality and Social Psychology, 38*, 909–923.

Wild, B., Erb, M., & Bartels, M. (2001). Are emotions contagious? Evoked emotions while viewing emotionally expressive faces: Quality, quantity, time course and gender differences. *Psychiatry Research, 102*, 109–124.

Wild, B., Erb, M., Eyb, M., Bartels, M., & Grodd, W. (2003). Why are smiles contagious? An fMRI study of the interaction between perception of facial affect and facial movements. *Psychiatry Research: Neuroimaging, 123*, 17–36.

Zajonc, R. B., Murphy, S. T., & Inglehart, M. (1989). Feeling and facial efference: Implications of the vascular theory of emotion. *Psychological Review, 96*, 395–416.

3   Being Imitated: Consequences of Nonconsciously Showing Empathy

Rick B. van Baaren, Jean Decety, Ap Dijksterhuis, Andries van der Leij, and
Matthijs L. van Leeuwen

To refrain from imitation is the best revenge.
—Marcus Aurelius, 121–180 AD

What is the relation between imitation and empathy? It is not an easy question to answer.
The crux of the problem is that there is no consensus on the definition of empathy.
Although most people intuitively "feel" what empathy means, its scientific study has a tur-
bulent past colored by a remarkable disagreement about its definition (see, for example,
Jahoda, 2005).

Empathy Lost in Translation

A look at the history of the debate over the definition of empathy makes clear why it is so
difficult to specify the relation between empathy and imitation. The word was translated
from English to German and back to English. It has moved back and forth between popular
usage, use in arts—such as aesthetics and drama—and use in the behavioral sciences. Finally,
it has suffered from the difficulty, common in psychology, of translating a subjective, intan-
gible, even hypothetical construct into words. Like a snowball rolling down a hill, the term
empathy has taken on association with a rather heterogeneous class of phenomena (for a
history, see Jahoda, 2005).

At the beginning of the twentieth century, before the term *empathy* was introduced, the
predecessors of this word (such as "sympathy" or the German *Einfühlung*) were sometimes
defined in terms of overt or covert motor imitation (e.g., Allport, 1968; Darwin, 1872/1965).
Theodor Lipps, for instance, touched upon the relation between empathy and imitation
when he described the process of *Einfühlung*: "When I see a gesture, there exists within
me a tendency to experience in myself the affect that naturally arises from that gesture.
And when there is no obstacle, the tendency is realized" (1907, quoted in Jahoda, 2005,
p. 719).

The middle and last decades of the twentieth century saw a shift toward the investigation
of "higher" levels of cognition, and the study of empathy followed suit. That is, during

these years, researchers paid more attention to strategic and conscious forms of empathy. However, recent theorizing once again gives motor imitation (mimicry) a prominent place in the process of empathy (e.g., Preston & De Waal, 2002; Decety & Jackson, 2004). Imitation is thought to play a mediating role; it is proposed that observers automatically mimic the behavior of a person they see. This elicits, through a proprioceptive process, a weaker version of the same state as the one which caused the target to behave. An example is emotional contagion, whereby a person automatically mimics someone's facial expression, resulting in a weaker version of the same emotion as that of the person being mimicked (Hatfield, Cacioppo, & Rapson, 1994).

Automaticity of Imitation

By now there is ample evidence for automatic imitation in humans. As the research in social psychology, developmental psychology, social neuroscience, and cognitive psychology has accumulated, many studies have shown how pervasive is our tendency to imitate. Imitation is observed in preverbal children (Meltzoff & Moore, 1977, 1997; though this finding has not gone unchallenged). People automatically and nonconsciously mimic the behaviors and mannerisms of their interaction partners, such as face-rubbing, touching one's hair, foot-shaking, and playing with a pen. In addition, laughter, yawning, mood, and various speech variables are known to be automatically imitated (Chartrand & Bargh, 1999; Van Baaren, Maddux, et al., 2003; Van Baaren, Horgan, et al., 2004).

The reason we mimic automatically is that the perception of a certain behavior automatically activates our own motor representation of that action (Decety & Chaminade, 2005; Iacoboni et al., 1999; Rizzolatti, Fogassi, & Gallese, 2001; Sommerville & Decety, 2006). In monkeys (macaques), single neurons have been identified in the premotor and posterior parietal cortices that fire both when a grasping hand movement is observed and when the monkey performs the grasping movement itself, illustrating a most intimate link between perception and action (Gallese et al., 1996). These neurons are now widely known as mirror neurons.

In humans, functionally similar effects have been observed, although not yet at the single-neuron level. For instance, perceiving hand movements activates the same cortical *region* in the ventral premotor cortex as performing that hand movement oneself (Iacoboni et al., 1999). Interestingly, a recent functional neuroimaging study shows that activity within the mirror system that results form viewing simple actions (i.e., grasping food) is modulated by the motivation (hungry vs. satiated) and goals of the perceiver (Cheng, Meltzoff, & Decety, 2006). According to some researchers, this "mirror neuron system" is responsible for imitation; however, no mediation of imitation by this putative mirror system has yet been documented. In sum, humans seem wired to imitate, and imitation is the default in the innumerable social interactions we have. But what role does imitation play in empathy?

Imitation and Empathy

In an attempt to create a framework integrating several views and phenomena related to empathy (including emotional contagion, sympathy, and cognitive empathy), Preston and De Waal (2002) postulated the perception-action model of empathy. Central to this model is the idea that empathy can best be described as a process. In this view, perception on an individual's state leads to activation of the perceiver's representation of that state and the situation, which subsequently activates the corresponding consequences and responses. The consequences can be cognitive, affective, behavioral, emotional, or a combination of these types. In this view, imitation and empathy are closely linked. Imitation is, in essence, the bridge leading to empathy. Indeed, developmental research indicates that we are hardwired for imitation with our conspecifics, and that such a mechanism is the stepping-stone to intersubjectivity (Meltzoff & Decety, 2003). Finally, recent research also shows that there is a correlation between a person's empathy and his or her tendency to imitate (Chartrand & Bargh, 1999; Dapretto et al., 2006).

The mechanism of imitation, the direct mapping of observed behavior onto our own behavioral representations, constitutes a rudimentary form of empathy because, in essence, imitation means that interaction partners have at least some of the same constructs or behavioral representations activated in the brain. Imitation, like empathy, requires overlap in cognition, feeling, and behavior. It is by no means a new idea to compare motor imitation with empathy. On one hand, the tendency to imitate is related to many indicators of prosociality, such as measures of rapport (e.g. Bavelas et al., 1987), empathy (Chartrand & Bargh, 1999), social or interdependent self-construal (Van Baaren, Maddux et al., 2003, Van Baaren, Horgan et al., 2004) and affiliation goals (Lakin & Chartrand, 2003). On the other hand, experimental work reveals that unobtrusive imitation results in positive interactions. Maurer and Tindall (1983), for example, looked at the effect of mimicry on perceived empathy in counselor-patient dyads. Their results indicated that when counselors mimicked the nonverbal behavior of the client, they were perceived as expressing more empathy compared to when the counselors did not mimic the client. Similarly, other researchers have described this type of motor mimicry as signaling feelings of similarity and understanding (e.g., Bavelas et al., 1987; Bernieri, 1988; LaFrance & Ickes, 1981; LaFrance, 1982).

At this point it is very important to note that the mimicry in all the research described in this chapter concerns *unobtrusive* mimicry. If someone consciously notices that you mimic their behavior, it will feel uncomfortable or can even be perceived as mockery (except in the case of very small children, who actually like seeing someone imitate them; Nadel, 2002). Normally, however, we are not aware of the mimicry that occurs in our daily interactions (Chartrand & Bargh, 1999).

Now that we know that we nonconsciously and automatically imitate others and that this similarity in cognition, feeling, and behavior is a form of empathy, the question arises, What exactly does being imitated do to us? In this chapter we want to elaborate on the *consequences* of showing empathy. Specifically, we will focus on motor imitation, because motor imitation means that someone behaves like you, which according to recent theorizing on empathy (e.g., Preston & de Waal, 2002) can be conceptualized as a nonconscious, low-level, or rudimentary form of empathy. What are the consequences of perceiving our own behavior mirrored by our interaction partner? Most of the available research has tackled this question by manipulating the amount of mimicry that occurs during social interactions, and then measuring the effect it has on self-report and behavior (for an overview, see Lakin & Chartrand, 2003).

Prosocial Effects of Being Imitated

In a typical experiment, a participant and a confederate are placed together in a room. The participants believe that they will work on a task, which in reality is an irrelevant task that is part of a cover story. During this bogus task, the confederate mimics the behavior of the participant. This mimicry occurs following a small delay, usually 3 or 4 seconds, and it is contralateral, mirroring the movement. Typical behaviors that are mimicked include face-rubbing, movements of the arms and legs, touching hair, etc. This "mimicry condition" is then contrasted with either a condition in which the participant is not mimicked by the confederate or (in some studies) with a condition where the confederate does the opposite of what the participant does.

Research using this general approach has shown that people who are imitated hold more positive views about a mimicking confederate than about a nonmimicking confederate. The above-mentioned study by Maurer and Tindall (1983), for example, showed an increase in perceived empathy. Chartrand and Bargh (1999) observed that people like mimickers better than nonmimickers and that they also rated the interaction as going more smoothly. Bailenson and Yee (2005) had a digital avatar in a virtual reality environment mimic (or not) the head movements of participants. This setting has the advantage of complete experimental control over behavior, and given the fact that avatars are computer generated, the effects cannot be explained by any form of experimenter expectancies or biases. Bailenson and Yee replicated the Chartrand and Bargh findings, indicating that it really is the act of unobtrusive mimicry that causes the more positive evaluations of the mimicker.

Because empathy also implies similarity between an actor and an observer, we recently conducted an experiment to test whether being mimicked actually does make you feel more similar to the mimicker (Van Baaren et al., 2007). After being imitated (or not) during an interaction, participants were asked to indicate how they felt about several opinion issues (e.g., there is too much nudity on television). In addition they were asked to indicate how they thought the experimenter felt about the same issues. This is a measure of projection: how much do you project your own thoughts and feelings onto someone else? (For a review, see Krueger & Robbins, 2005.) The results revealed more projection after mimicry, which means that mimicry makes people feel more similar. Thus, mimicry affects how we *judge* our interaction partner. Does it also affect how we *behave* toward him or her?

In the last few years, several researchers have investigated the behavioral consequences of imitation. If it really is a "social glue"(Dijksterhuis, 2005; Lakin, et al., 2003), that smoothes interactions and fosters bonding in humans, these effects should be observed on a behavioral level: imitation should "pay off." In a very literal test of this premise, Van Baaren, Holland, et al., (2003) instructed waitresses in a restaurant in the Netherlands to either verbally mimic customers when ordering, or to merely paraphrase the order. It is known that people mimic all sorts of speech variables (Giles & Coupland, 1991; Gregory, Dagan, & Webster, 1997), making this type of mimicry ideally suited for use as an independent imitation variable. Afterward, the amount of tips the waitress received was assessed to see whether mimicry increases tipping. In the two studies of this type, the results showed a significant difference (of more than 50%) between the amount of tips received in the mimicry and the no-mimicry condition; mimicry literally did pay off.

Despite its ecological validity, an unpredictable and relatively uncontrolled restaurant setting is not ideal for experimentally testing the behavioral effects of mimicry. Therefore, we conceptually replicated the restaurant findings in a more controlled laboratory environment. In this experiment (Van Baaren, Holland, et al., 2004, Study 1), participants were mimicked or not by an experimenter while they were working on a bogus "marketing task." When the task was over, the experimenter said that the experiment had finished and that he would leave the room the get some material for an unrelated experiment. After approximately one minute, he reentered the room carrying some papers with ten pens on top. Directly after entering the room he "accidentally" tripped, dropping the pens on the floor. This procedure was borrowed from Macrae and Johnston (1998). The dependent variable was the helpfulness of the participant: would the participant start to help the experimenter? The results showed a strong effect of mimicry: mimicked participants were more likely to help the experimenter, thereby conceptually replicating the restaurant findings in a controlled environment.

There is a confound in all of these studies on being imitated, which lies in the fact that the dependent variable is always related to the mimicker: Do you like the mimicker more? Do you help her more often? This method makes it impossible to say whether the effects of mimicry hold only for the mimicker, or whether the effects of mimicry are more general. Does mimicry create a special bond between two interaction partners? Or does being mimicked affect a person more profoundly? Does it change not only how we judge and behave toward the mimicker, but also toward other, even unrelated, others?

Several recent studies have addressed this question. Van Baaren and colleagues, for example, replicated the experiment discussed previously on helpfulness (i.e., the one whereby participants picked up pens), but this time they manipulated whether a confederate unrelated to the mimicry study dropped the pens (Van Baaren, Holland, et al., 2004). After the mimicry was manipulated by the first (female) experimenter, she told the participants that she would leave the room and a new experimenter would give instructions for a new and unrelated experiment. When that new experimenter entered the room, she "accidentally" dropped the pens on the floor. Again, mimicked participants were more helpful than nonmimicked participants, suggesting a broader prosocial effect of mimicry. To ensure that this effect was not driven by similarity between the mimicker and the new person, a third study measured helpfulness toward an abstract entity: A charity. After the mimicry manipulation, the participants were paid and either the same or a new experimenter told the participants that the university conducted research for the CliniClowns (a well-known charity in the Netherlands). Participants were asked to complete an anonymous questionnaire and were told there was an opportunity to donate money. Subsequently, the experimenter left the room, leaving the participant alone in a room with a questionnaire and a sealed collecting box. For the participants, the donating behavior was completely anonymous.

Did mimicry increase donations? Indeed it did, and it did so irrespective of whether the experimenter was the same as in the mimicry experiment or a new one. These data strongly suggest that mimicry affects us in a way that goes beyond building a special bond with the mimicker. It make us generally more prosocial as people. More evidence for this increased prosociality is found in a recent paper by Ashton-James and colleagues (2007). In several studies, they demonstrated how being imitated makes people feel more close and connected to other people. In addition, mimicked participants also actually sit closer to unknown others, that is, their preferred interpersonal distance is decreased.

Cognitive Style

The research discussed in the previous section shows that being imitated has important social consequences. We become more helpful, and, in general, being mimicked makes us more sociable. Because being imitated deeply affects how we interact with our environment, we may also find effects on a fundamental perceptual level. That is, do we only behave differently, or do we also perceive the world in a different way as a result of being mimicked?

Some researchers have looked at the relation between being mimicked and "cognitive style." Cognitive styles describe the ways that individuals perceive, organize, and respond to stimuli, in other words, the "form" or "process" rather than the "content" or "level" of cognition (Witkin & Goodenough, 1977). One of the most extensively investigated individual differences in cognitive style has been that of field dependence versus field independence. Witkin, Goodenough, and Oltman (1979) have argued that individuals with a field-dependent cognitive style tend to rely more on "external referents" (i.e., contextual cues) than do field-independent individuals across of variety of domains, from perception to interpersonal behavior.

As applied to visual perception, field dependence involves integrating objects and their respective contexts, whereas field independence involves differentiating between the focal object and its field, or context. Field dependence can be measured in several different ways—for example, with the Hidden Figures Test (Witkin et al., 1971). In this test, participants see several complex geometrical objects. Within these complex shapes, simple geometrical objects, such as a square or triangle, are "hidden." The task of the participants is to detect the simple object. Field independence enhances performance on this task, because it helps the participant to focus on details and ignore the disturbance by the context. When you are field independent, you are less distracted by the complex shape, making it easier for you to detect the embedded figure. In contrast, a field-dependent style leads to more difficulty in isolating and detecting the simple object amid the complex figure.

There is a strong relation between cognitive style and interpersonal behavior. Compared to field-independent individuals, field-dependent individuals show more attentiveness to social cues (Fitzgibbons, Goldberger, & Eagle, 1965; Rajecki, Ickes, & Tanford, 1981) and a greater tendency to be influenced by others (e.g., Gul, Huang, & Subramaniam, 1992; Rajecki, Ickes, & Tanford, 1981).

Given this relation between cognitive style and the social aspects of interpersonal behavior on the one hand, and the social consequences of being imitated on the other hand, we tested whether being imitated makes us more field dependent (Van Baaren, Horgan, et al., 2004). First, participants were imitated or not, then they were given a memory task designed by Kuhnen and Oyserman (2002; see also Chalfonte & Johnson, 1996), which measures context dependency in information processing. In this task, participants were instructed to look carefully at a sheet of paper consisting of 28 randomly located simple objects (e.g., house, rose, piano). After 90 seconds, the experimenter replaced the sheet with another piece of paper containing an empty grid and said the following. "Now I would like you to remember what you have just seen. Please try to remember what you have seen and where you have seen it. Write down in the cells of this grid the items you saw in the place you saw each one. If you can remember an item, but not where it was, you can write it down outside the grid. Please try to remember as many items and their positions as possible." In this task, a more context-dependent information processing style was inferred from higher scores, that is, from a better memory for the correct locations of the viewed objects.

The results clearly showed increased field dependence after imitation. In both conditions, participants remembered an equal amount of objects. In the imitation condition however, people were 50% better at indicating the correct location. It appears that being imitated leads to a field-dependent processing style. Together with the data on prosocial behavior and interpersonal closeness, this finding provides strong evidence for the idea that being imitated does not just lead to a special bond between the mimicker and mimickee. Instead, it profoundly affects how one perceives and interacts with the (social) environment.

The Social Neuroscience of Being Imitated

Finally, an interesting question concerns the neurological underpinnings of these forms of unobtrusive mimicry. How does our brain detect it? Note that we are not aware of being imitated, but it still affects us. What does this nonconscious imitation recognition look like? What are the neural correlates of being imitated? To date, all neuroscience research on the neural mechanisms underpinning imitation has investigated intentional tasks (see Decety, 2006, for a recent review).

Based on the research we have described on the consequences of imitation, several hypotheses can be proposed. Interestingly, although the effects and consequences of mimicry are always reported in comparison to nonmimicry conditions, the largest effects are actually seen in the nonmimicry condition (e.g., see Van Baaren, Maddux, et al., 2003) and the mimicry condition often resembles a control condition. Being imitated seems to be the default.

One could therefore hypothesize that not being imitated (rather than being imitated) is experienced as being unexpected. This may lead to negative affect and therefore tap into neural systems that process negative affect, including the anterior insula (e.g., Phan et al., 2002) and the part of the anterior cingulate cortex that deals with conflict monitoring (e. g., Kerns et al., 2004). In essence this is how the German philosophers in the beginning of the twentieth century conceptualized *Einfühlung*. Lipps (1907 in Jahoda, 2005), in comparing *Einfühlung* with the law of gravity, theorized that it is not the occurrence, but the absence, that calls for an explanation.

Advanced neuroimaging techniques present expanded opportunities to study the consequences of imitation, but there are practical problems as well. Two major obstacles that hinder such work with functional magnetic resonance imaging (fMRI) are the very restricted possibilities of moving while in the scanner and the difficulty of making imitation go unnoticed. In a recent pilot study, we tested a paradigm to circumvent these problems. In an fMRI scanner, participants were asked to imagine either a very sad event in their lives, a neutral event, or a very happy event, and to adopt the corresponding facial expression. Then we subliminally flashed either happy, sad, or neutral faces to produce congruent and incongruent perception-action pairings (that is, imitative and opposite facial expressions). The results were encouraging: The incongruent conditions showed the expected activation of areas related to expectancy violation or conflict and self-other distinction (anterior cingulate cortex and temporal parietal junction). It may be the case that the absence of imitation is unexpected and perceived as negative. Although these data are only preliminary, they suggest a promising line of research.

Conclusion

Imitation is an important facet of empathy: it fosters similarity in behavior, cognition, and feeling. Our review of work on the consequences of this rudimentary form of empathy makes it clear that—despite going unnoticed—imitation has profound effects on the way we perceive and interact with our social environment. It makes us more prosocial and seems to function as "social glue" (Dijksterhuis, 2005; Lakin et al., 2003). In fact, it seems that the condition of *not* being imitated has the greater impact on behavior. People expect others to think like them, behave like them, and feel like them. As the Roman emperor Marcus Aurelius knew, empathy is the default, and the absence of empathy is painful.

References

Allport, G. (1968). The historical background of modern social psychology. In G. Lindzey & E. Aronson (Eds.), *Handbook of social psychology*. Reading, MA: Addison-Wesley.

Ashton-James, C., Van Baaren, R. B., Chartrand, T. L., & Decety, J. (2007). Mimicry and me: The impact of mimicry on self-construal. *Social Cognition, 25,* 518–535.

Bailenson, J., & Yee, N. (2005). Digital Chameleons: Automatic assimilation of nonverbal gestures in immersive virtual environments. *Psychological Science, 16,* 814-819.

Bavelas, J. B., Black, A., Lemery, C. R., & Mullett, J. (1987). Motor mimicry as primitive empathy. In N. Eisenberg & J. Strayer (Eds.), *Empathy and its development* (pp. 317–338). Cambridge: Cambridge University Press.

Bernieri, F. J. (1988). Coordinated movement and rapport in teacher-student interactions. *Journal of Nonverbal Behavior, 12,* 120–138.

Chalfonte, B. L., & Johnson, M. K. (1996). Feature memory and binding in young and older adults. *Memory and Cognition, 24,* 403–416.

Chartrand, T. L., & Bargh, J. A. (1999). The chameleon effect: The perception-behavior link and social interaction. *Journal of Personality and Social Psychology, 76,* 893–910.

Cheng, Y., Meltzoff, A. N., & Decety, J. (2007). Motivation modulates the activity of the human mirror system: An fMRI study. *Cerebral Cortex, 17,* 1979–1986.

Dapretto, M., Davies, M., Pfeifer, J., Scott, A., Sigman, M., Bookheimer., S., & Iacoboni, M. (2006). Understanding emotions in others: Mirror neuron dysfunction in children with autism spectrum disorder. *Nature Neuroscience, 6,* 28–30.

Darwin, C. (1872/1965). *The expression of the emotions in man and animals.* Chicago: University of Chicago Press.

Decety, J. (2006). A cognitive neuroscience view of imitation. In S. Rogers & J. Williams (Eds.), *Imitation and the social mind: Autism and typical development* (pp. 251–274). New York: Guilford Press.

Decety, J., & Chaminade, T. (2005). The neurophysiology of imitation and intersubjectivity. In S. Hurley & N. Chater (Eds.), *Perspectives on imitation: From neuroscience to social science: Vol. 1. Mechanisms of imitation and imitation in animals* (pp. 119–140). Cambridge, MA: MIT press.

Decety, J., & Jackson, P. L. (2004). The functional architecture of human empathy. *Behavioral and Cognitive Neuroscience Reviews, 3,* 71–100.

Dijksterhuis, A. (2005). Why we are social animals: The high road to imitation as social glue. In S. Hurley & N. Chater (Eds.), *Perspectives on imitation: From cognitive neuroscience to social science: Vol. 2. Imitation, human development, and culture* (pp. 207–220). Cambridge, MA: MIT Press.

Fitzgibbons, D., Goldberger, L., & Eagle, M. (1965). Field dependence and memory for incidental material. *Perceptual and Motor Skills, 21*, 743–749.

Gallese, V., Fadiga, L., Fogassi, L., & Rizzolatti, G. (1996). Action recognition in the premotor cortex. *Brain, 119*, 593–609.

Giles, H., & Coupland, N. (1991). *Language: Context and consequences.* Milton Keynes, UK: Open University Press.

Gregory, S. W., Dagan, K., & Webster, S. (1997). Evaluating the relation of vocal accommodation in conversation partners' fundamental frequencies to perceptions of communication quality. *Journal of Nonverbal Behavior, 21*, 23–43.

Gul, F., Huang, A., & Subramaniam, N. (1992). Cognitive style as a factor in accounting students' perceptions of career-choice factors. *Psychological Reports, 71*, 1275–1281.

Hatfield, E., Cacioppo, J., & Rapson, R. (1994). *Emotional contagion.* Cambridge: Cambridge University Press.

Iacoboni, M. (2005). Understanding others: Imitation, language, and empathy. In S. Hurley & N. Chater (Eds.), *Perspectives on imitation: From neuroscience to social science: Vol. 1. Mechanisms of imitation and imitation in animals* (pp. 77–99). Cambridge: MIT Press.

Iacoboni, M., Woods, R., Brass, M., Bekkering, H., Mazziotta, J. C., & Rizzolatti, G. (1999). Cortical mechanisms of human imitation. *Science, 286*, 2526–2528.

Jahoda, G. (2005). Theodor Lipps and the shift from "sympathy" to "empathy." *Journal of the History of the Behavioral Sciences, 41*, 151–163.

Kerns, J. G., Cohen, J. D., MacDonall, A. W., Cho, R. Y., Stenger, V. A., & Carter, C. S. (2004). Anterior cingulate conflict monitoring and adjustments in control. *Science, 303*, 1023–1026.

Krueger, J., & Robbins, J. M. (2005). Social Projection to Ingroups and Outgroups: A review and meta-analysis. *Personality and Social Psychology Review, 9* (1), 32–47.

Kuhnen, U., & Oyserman, D. (2002). Thinking about the self influences thinking in general: Cognitive consequences of salient self-concept. *Journal of Experimental Psychology, 38*, 492-499.

LaFrance, M. (1982). Posture mirroring and rapport. In M. Davis (Ed.), *Interaction rhythms: Periodicity in communicative behavior* (pp. 279–298). New York: Human Sciences Press.

LaFrance, M., & Ickes, W. (1981). Posture mirroring and interactional involvement: Sex and sex typing effects. *Journal of Nonverbal Behavior, 5, 139–154.*

Lakin, J., & Chartrand, T. L. (2003). Increasing nonconscious mimicry to achieve rapport. *Psychological Science, 27*, 145–162.

Lakin, J. L., Jefferis, V., Cheng, C. M., & Chartrand, T. L. (2003). The chameleon effect as social glue: Evidence for the evolutionary significance of nonconscious mimicry. *Journal of Nonverbal Behavior, 27*, 145–157.

Macrae, C. N., & Johnston, L. (1998). Help, I need somebody: Automatic action and inaction. *Social Cognition, 16,* 400–417.

Maurer, R., & Tindall, J. (1983). Effect of postural congruence on client's perception of counselor empathy. *Journal of Counseling Psychology, 30,* 158–163.

Meltzoff, A. (1990). Foundations for developing a concept of self: The role of imitation in relating self to other and the value of social mirroring, social modeling, and self-practice in infancy. In D. Cicchetti & M. Beeghly (Eds.), *The self in transition* (pp. 139–164). Chicago: University of Chicago Press.

Meltzoff, A. N., & Decety, J. (2003). What imitation tells us about social cognition: A rapprochement between developmental psychology and cognitive neuroscience. *Philosophical Transactions of the Royal Society, London, B, 358,* 491–500.

Meltzoff, A. N., & Moore, M. K. (1977). Imitation of facial and manual gestures by human neonates. *Science, 198,* 75–78.

Meltzoff, A. N., & Moore, M. K. (1997). Explaining facial imitation: A theoretical model. *Early development and parenting, 6,* 179–192.

Nadel, J. (2002). Imitation and imitation recognition: Functional use in preverbal infants and nonverbal children with autism. In A. Meltzoff & W. Prinz (Eds.), *The imitative mind* (pp. 42–62). Cambridge: Cambridge University Press.

Phan, K. L., Wager, T., Taylor, S. F., & Liberzon, I. (2002). Functional neuroanatomy of emotion: A meta-analysis of emotion activations studies in PET and fMRI. *NeuroImage, 16,* 331–348.

Preston, S., & de Waal, F. (2002). Empathy: Its ultimate and proximate bases. *Behavioral and Brain Sciences, 25,* 1–72.

Rajecki, D., Ickes, W., & Tanford, S. (1981). Locus of control and reactions to a stranger. *Personality and Social Psychology Bulletin, 7,* 139–154.

Rizzolatti, G., Fogassi, L., & Gallese, V. (2001). Neurophysiological mechanisms underlying action understanding and imitation. *Nature Reviews Neuroscience, 2,* 661–670.

Schall, J. D. (2001). Neural basis of deciding, choosing and acting. *Nature Reviews Neuroscience, 2,* 33–42.

Shipman, S., & Shipman, V. C. (1985). Cognitive styles: Some conceptual, methodological, and applied issues. In E. Gordon (Ed.), *Review of research in education* (pp. 229–291). Washington, DC: American Educational Research Association.

Sommerville, J. A., & Decety, J. (2006). Weaving the fabric of social interaction: Articulating developmental psychology and cognitive neuroscience in the domain of motor cognition. *Psychonomic Bulletin and Review, 13* (2), 179–200.

Tiedens, L., & Fragale, A. (2003). Power moves: Complementarity in dominant and submissive nonverbal behavior. *Journal of Personality and Social Psychology, 84,* 558–568.

Van Baaren, R. B., Ames, D., Vossen, R., Jones, P., & Dijksterhuis, A. (2008). *Projection and imitation*. Manuscript submitted for publication.

Van Baaren, R. B., Holland, R. W., Kawakami, K., & van Knippenberg, A. (2004). Mimicry and pro-social behavior. *Psychological Science, 15,* 71–74.

Van Baaren, R. B., Holland, R. W., Steenaert, B., & van Knippenberg, A. (2003). Mimicry for money: Behavioral consequences of imitation. *Journal of Experimental Social Psychology, 39,* 393–398.

Van Baaren, R. B., Horgan, T. G., Chartrand, T. L., & Dijkmans, M. (2004). The forest, the trees and the chameleon: Context-dependency and mimicry. *Journal of Personality and Social Psychology, 86,* 453–459.

Van Baaren, R. B., Maddux, W. W., Chartrand, T. L., de Bouter, C., & van Knippenberg, A. (2003). It takes two to mimic: Behavioral consequences of self-construals. *Journal of Personality and Social Psychology, 84,* 1093–1102.

Witkin, H. A., & Goodenough, D. R. (1977). Field dependence and interpersonal behavior. *Psychological Bulletin, 84,* 661–689.

Witkin, H. A., Goodenough, D. R., & Oltman, P. K. (1979). Psychological differentiation: Current status. *Journal of Personality and Social Psychology, 37,* 1127–1145.

Witkin, H. A., Oltman, P. K., Raskin, E., & Karp, S. A. (1971). *A manual for the embedded figures tests*. Palo Alto, CA: Consulting Psychologists Press.

4 Empathy and Knowledge Projection

Raymond S. Nickerson, Susan F. Butler, and Michael Carlin

The word *empathy* conveys the notion of shared or vicarious feeling; to empathize with another is to imagine oneself in the other's situation and to experience, to some degree, the emotions that the other is experiencing. For the purposes of this chapter, we note that the concept has also a more cognitive aspect, which is made explicit in the following definition from Webster's *New Collegiate Dictionary*: "the capacity for participation in another's feelings *or ideas*" (emphasis ours). Our interest is in the question of how we form beliefs about what others feel and know, and to what extent the answer can be found in what we ourselves feel and know. Our hypothesis is that people's ability to empathize—to participate in another's feelings and ideas—is based, at least in part, on people's tendency to impute to others their own feelings and knowledge. This idea, or something close to it, has many proponents (Fussell & Krauss, 1991; Hodges & Wegner, 1997; Karniol, 1990; Krueger, 1998; Nickerson, 1999; O'Mahony, 1984; Royzman, Cassidy, & Baron, 2003).

Necessity of Judging What Others Know

If we did not make judgments of what other people know, how they feel, and what they are likely to do in specific situations, communication would be impossible. Writers have to gauge their expositions to the level of relevant background knowledge expected of their intended audiences. Speakers in everyday conversation must make assumptions about what the other parties to the conversation do and do not know in order to ensure that what they say will be understood.

Researchers who study the performance of work teams emphasize the importance of the team members having similar mental models of the processes and situations with which they have to deal corporately (Rouse, Cannon-Bowers, & Salas, 1992), especially when performing under stressful conditions (Cannon-Bowers, Salas, & Converse, 1993). When people collaborate in real time at a distance, as for example when using software ("groupware") intended to facilitate such collaboration, it is important that each collaborator have a reasonably accurate understanding of what the others are doing and thinking (Gutwin & Greenberg, 2002). When one performs as a member of an interacting team, adequate awareness of one's situation may include awareness of one's teammates' perception of the situation and of their knowledge of what must be done (Andersen, Pedersen, & Andersen, 2001).

A major basis for such judgments and assumptions is what one oneself knows, and what one believes about how one would feel or what one would do in the situations of interest. Collingwood (1946) makes the point that both the historian, writing about actions and feelings of people of the past, and readers, attempting to understand history, can make sense of it all only by imagining how they would react in the circumstances described. Steedman and Johnson-Laird (1980) suggest that in conversation "the speaker assumes that the hearer knows everything that the speaker knows about the world and about the conversation, unless there is some evidence to the contrary" (p. 129). O'Mahony (1984) argues that projection is a basic mode of knowing other persons, and that projective effects are likely to be the more pronounced the less one knows about another onto whom one's own characteristics are being projected.

The argument has been made that one's knowledge or belief about how one would behave or react in specific situations can be a useful basis, possibly the best basis one has, for anticipating how other people will behave or react in those situations (Dawes, 1989; Hoch, 1987; Krueger & Zeiger, 1993; Nickerson, 1999). This idea is captured in the "principle of humanity," according to which when trying to understand what someone has said, especially something ambiguous, one should impute to the speaker beliefs and desires similar to one's own (Gordon, 1986; Grandy, 1973). And there is reason to believe that, under certain conditions, people who project their own opinions to others may predict other people's opinions more accurately than those who do not (Stanovich & West, 1998).

Reflection: Projection in Reverse

The assumption that other people are much like oneself—or, equivalently, that one is much like others—provides a basis for inferences either way: from oneself to others or from others to oneself. Our interest is primarily in projection from oneself to others, and the bulk of this chapter addresses that, but we note first some evidence that inferences occur also in the opposite direction. We will refer to this phenomenon as *reflection*—projection in reverse.

What people know or believe about others' knowledge or abilities can influence how they perceive their own (Valins & Nisbett, 1972; Weiner et al., 1972). Several investigators have shown, for example, that in the absence of direct experiential evidence of their own ability to perform specific tasks, people sometimes judge that ability on the basis of what they know or believe about the abilities of those in a peer or reference group (Bandura, 1982; Gist & Mitchell, 1992).

Nelson and colleagues (1986) found that for general-knowledge questions that people could not answer directly, normative item difficulty (accuracy base rates) better predicted their ability to recognize the answers than did their own "feeling of knowing" ratings of the unrecalled answers. Calogero and Nelson (1992) gave some participants base-rate information (telling them the percentage of people in the database who knew the answer) regarding each question they could not answer. Relative to participants who did not get the base-rate information, those who did gave higher feeling-of-knowing ratings for the normatively easier questions than for the normatively difficult ones. One interpretation of this outcome is that participants' own feeling of knowing changed in the direction of what they had learned about what others know. Another is that they simply adjusted their reports of feeling of knowing so as to be more consistent with the normative data. Either way, the normative information was "helpful" to the participants in that they became more confident that they would recognize the answers to those questions whose answers they were, in fact, more likely to identify correctly.

Evidence of Projection

The hypothesis that people project their own feelings, opinions, attitudes, judgments, behaviors, desires, and so on to others was entertained by certain psychologists several decades ago (Cattell, 1944; Katz & Allport, 1931; Wallen, 1943) and has received a great deal of empirical support (Krueger, 1998). Since the time of Katz and Allport's discovery that students who admitted to cheating on exams were more likely than those who did not to expect others to cheat as well, many studies have verified that people who engage in a particular behavior tend to estimate that behavior to be more prevalent than do people who do not engage in it (Marks & Miller, 1987; Mullen, 1983; Ross, Greene, & House, 1977).

Other experimental results demonstrate our tendency to view ourselves as representative of other people in specific respects:

· How happy one perceives others to be depends in part on how happy one considers oneself to be (Goldings, 1954).
· Victims of crime tend to make higher estimates of the incidence of crime than do people who have not been victims (Bennett & Hibberd, 1986).
· People's judgments of how difficult anagram problems are likely to be for others correlate highly with the solution times for themselves (Jacoby & Kelley, 1987).
· After hearing 50 actors express opinions on a controversial issue, college students estimated the distribution of the actors' opinions to favor their own prior positions, although the distribution was, in fact, evenly divided on the issue (Kassin, 1981).

Recent data from our own laboratory supplement these findings. In one experiment (whose results essentially replicated those of a previous study by Nickerson, Baddeley, and Freeman, 1987), estimates by college students of the percentage of peers who would know answers to general-knowledge questions increased according to their confidence in their own answers to the questions, and this was true both for questions the participants answered correctly and those they answered incorrectly.

In a second experiment, students attempted to provide the names of the capital cities of U.S. states and of various foreign countries. They gave a confidence rating for each response and then estimated the percentage of their peers who would produce the correct name. (Other conditions were also used that are not reported here.) Again, the estimated percentage of peers who would produce the correct answer was positively correlated with the participants' confidence that they had produced the correct answer, and this effect was evident when their answers were incorrect as well as when they were correct.

In a third experiment, students were given several problems to solve. An example: "Arrange 10 dots in such a way that there are 5 rows with 4 dots in each row (a row being a set of dots through which one can draw a straight line). A single dot may appear in 2 rows but not more than 2 rows." Participants attempted to solve the problems themselves, and they estimated the percentage of their peers who would be able to solve them. The pattern of results was generally consistent with the hypothesis that people who can solve a problem are more likely than those who cannot to assume that others will be able to solve it too.

In the final experiment of this series, students estimated the number of items in each of several categories (chemical elements, Shakespeare's plays, NBA teams, etc.) that they could list in 15 minutes and then estimated the number of items in each of the same categories that their peers could list, on average, in the same amount of time. Of interest was the question of whether, *for individual categories,* there would be a positive correlation between people's estimates for themselves and their estimates for others. Such a correlation should be found if people tend to assume that others are likely to know what they themselves know. We hypothesized that, on average, people who believe they themselves could list a relatively large number of names of chemical elements, say, are likely to give higher estimates of how many names of elements others can list than are those who believe they themselves could list few such names. Results bore out this expectation. Pearson *r* correlation coefficients for self and other estimates for the 18 categories ranged from a low of .41 for chemical elements to a high of .94 for mammals; the median correlation was .77.

A Statistical Case for Projection

A case can be made that projection should provide some advantage in guessing for strictly statistical reasons. Suppose that 80 percent of a specified population knows that Grover Cleveland served two nonconsecutive terms as president of the United States and 20 percent does not know this. Suppose further that those who know the fact assume that *everyone* in the population does, and that those who do not know it assume that *nobody* does. Eighty percent of the population (the 80 percent that knows the fact) will be right in their imputation of this knowledge to others 80 percent of the time, and the 20 percent that does not know it will be right in assuming that others do not know 20 percent of the time. So, over the entire population, the probability that a random person will correctly impute knowledge, or lack of knowledge, of this fact to a random other person will be

Table 4.1
Probability of correct imputation of knowledge (or lack thereof) depending on prevalence of knowledge within the group

Percentage with knowledge	Probability of correct imputation
0 or 100	1.00
10 or 90	.82
20 or 80	.68
30 or 70	.58
40 or 60	.52
50	.50

$(0.8 \times 0.8) + (0.2 \times 0.2) = 0.68$. One gets the same result if one starts with the assumption that only 20 percent knows the fact and 80 percent does not know it: $(0.2 \times 0.2) + (0.8 \times 0.8) = 0.68$. The probability that a random member of the group would be correct in imputing his or her own knowledge (or lack thereof) of the fact regarding Cleveland to a random other member of the group is shown in table 4.1. As the table illustrates, projecting assures that the guesser won't be wrong more than half the time in a binary situation.

Common-Ground Assumptions in Communication

One aspect of what it means to be a competent language user is the ability to use common ground—a shared context—in referential communication (Clark & Haviland, 1977; Clark & Marshall, 1981). But success in conversation depends not only on the existence of common ground but on each participant's knowledge of what the common ground is, their knowledge that they share it, and each one's knowledge that the other is aware of this (Clark & Carlson, 1981). The ability to use common ground effectively is one that children acquire gradually during their formative years (Ackerman, Szymanski, & Silver, 1990; Deutsch & Pechmann, 1982).

According to the *audience design* hypothesis, speakers design messages to be appropriate to the knowledge they assume the recipients of those messages have (Clark & Murphy, 1982; Clark, Schreuder, & Buttrick, 1983; Fussell & Krauss, 1992). An opposing view is represented by a *monitoring and adjustment* or *perspective adjustment* model of language comprehension, according to which language users do not plan utterances with the assumed knowledge of recipients in mind, but rely on common ground to correct errors of comprehension (Horton & Keysar, 1996; Keysar et al., 1998). This model assumes, for example, that when a listener has to find a referent for a definite reference (*the* boy, as distinct from *a* boy) a search that is not restricted to common-ground referents is initiated. During this search, and more or less simultaneously, a slower comprehension-monitoring process that is sensitive to common ground gets under way and makes an adjustment, if necessary, to ensure comprehension. The audience-design and adjustment models differ in important respects, but both recognize one's knowledge of others' knowledge as an important component of effective communication.

Presumably, we all have some notion of what is encompassed by the phrase "common knowledge," but it is an imprecise concept with fuzzy boundaries. What do we mean when we say that something is common knowledge? Knowledge that everyone has? Knowledge that (nearly) everyone (in a specific, but not necessarily specified, population) has?

Clearly we recognize different degrees of commonness; we expect some things to be known by a larger percentage of people than others. Some things we all know by virtue of being human beings (for example, that we all require sleep). Some things can be assumed to be known by all, or most, members of the same culture, inhabitants of the same geographical region, graduates of the same school, members of the same family, and so on. The problem of judging what others know is most interesting somewhere between the extremes—where some people, but not all, can be assumed to be "in the know."

One generally assumes:

• That a resident of a town knows more about that town than does a non-resident.
• That an automobile mechanic knows more about cars than does the average driver.
• That a cancer survivor has a better understanding of what it is like to face a life-threatening illness than does a person who has always enjoyed good health.

It follows that models of others' knowledge that are based solely on one's own knowledge are likely to need some degree of adjustment on the basis of individuating information if they are to avoid being inaccurate in many particulars. Such knowledge is acquired in many ways, but perhaps especially through direct, person-to-person interaction. As the monitoring-and-adjustment model of language comprehension has it, one may discover in conversation that a particular assumption about shared knowledge is not valid and therefore must be modified. When there is doubt as to what another person knows that is relevant to an interaction, direct probing—"Do you know anything about . . .?" "Are you from this area?"—may suffice to effect the necessary change in one's model of what the other knows.

Projection Can Also Fail

We have argued that the projection of one's own knowledge, feelings, and behavior to others is necessary and useful and have reviewed evidence that it occurs. We should also recognize that projection can, and often does, fail. In assuming that another random individual has much in common with oneself, one can be wrong in either of two ways: the degree of commonality that is assumed may be either more or less than actually pertains. The available evidence suggests that people are more likely to overestimate than to underestimate what others know on a subject with which they themselves are familiar, in part because of uncritical imputation of their own knowledge of that subject to others. In short, we tend to overproject—to view ourselves as more representative of other people in specific respects than we really are.

• Voters tend to overestimate the popularity of their favored candidate in a presidential election (Granberg & Brent, 1974, 1983).
• People are likely to overestimate the amount of consensus on their own opinions and to underestimate the amount on opinions they do not hold (Kassin, 1979; Ross, Green, & House, 1977).
• Inexperienced writers characteristically overestimate the degree to which their intended audience shares their own values and perspective (Hayes et al., 1987).
• Reviewers of journal manuscripts tend to overestimate the extent to which other reviews will agree with their own (Mahoney, 1977).
• Children often assume that another person sees a visual scene from the same perspective as they do, even though the other person is viewing it from a different angle or location (cf. Pufall & Shaw, 1973).

We have found, in experiments briefly mentioned above, that people are likely to project not only what they know but also what they erroneously believe they know: the level of confidence in one's own knowledge was consistently a strong predictor of the probability of projecting, whether or not the confidence was justified.

Jacoby, Bjork, and Kelley (1994) refer to the tendency to overproject as a form of egocentrism and describe it this way: "[P]eople engage in a form of egocentrism when they fail to realize that their subjective experience of the difficulty of a problem, the comprehensibility of a text, or the ease of learning a task may not generalize to other people's experience of the problem, text, or task. . . . [P]eople are surprisingly insensitive to the ways their construal of a particular situation is idiosyncratic" (p. 59).

Appropriately gauging the knowledge of one's audience can be a considerable challenge to a lecturer or writer. It is relatively easy for an expert in a particular area to address other experts in the same area. What is more difficult is to write or speak informatively, but not condescendingly, for readers or listeners who are not expert in the subject area. Piaget (1962) recognized how difficult it is for teachers, especially beginning teachers, to see things from the perspectives of their students. "Every beginning instructor discovers sooner or later that his first lectures were incomprehensible because he was talking to himself, so to say, mindful only of his own point of view. He realizes only gradually and with difficulty that it is not easy to place oneself in the shoes of students who do not know what he knows about the subject matter of his course" (quoted in Jacoby, Bjork, & Kelley, 1994, p. 63).

Flavell (1977) makes the same point from the perspective of a student: "[T]he fact that you thoroughly understand calculus constitutes an obstacle to your continuously keeping in mind my ignorance of it while trying to explain it to me; you may momentarily realize how hard it is for me, but that realization may quietly slip away once you get immersed in your explanation" (p. 124).

The ease with which an expert can overestimate the accessibility to others of his own expertise is suggested by a comment once made by the famous polymath Henri Poincaré (reported in Henle, 1962, p. 35). "How does it happen that there are people who do not understand mathematics? . . . There is nothing mysterious in the fact that everyone is not capable of discovery. . . . But what does seem most surprising, when we consider it, is that anyone should be unable to understand a mathematical argument at the very moment it is stated to him." We suspect that we all tend to underestimate how difficult other people will find it to grasp ideas with which we have been familiar for a long time.

A compelling case of overprojection was demonstrated by Newton (1990), who had some participants in an experiment tap rhythms of well-known songs while other participants tried to identify the songs to which the rhythms belonged. Tappers expected listeners to identify about half of the songs; in fact they correctly identified only about 1 in 40. It is surprisingly easy for one who has privileged knowledge (the tapper in this case) to project that knowledge to one who does not have it (the listener). The reader may wish to try this experiment informally. As one taps a rhythm, one may find it hard to believe that the song from which it comes, which one "hears" as one taps, is not immediately obvious to the listener. Of course, in performing the experiment, one has to be careful not to convey clues of the song other than its rhythm.

If one finds it easy to do X, one is likely to assume that others too should find it easy to do X; and, similarly, if doing X is difficult for oneself, one is likely to assume that it will be difficult for others as well. When Person A describes something to Person B, it is very easy for Person A to assume, even without realizing that she is doing so, that Person B is seeing in his mind's eye just what she sees in hers, as she is describing it. Who has not had the experience of being given "you-can't-miss-it" directions by a resident of a town that one is visiting, and finding them impossible to follow, or perhaps even to comprehend? Our conjecture is that the person giving directions has knowledge of the layout of the area—a mental map—and she, in effect, overlooks the fact that the recipient of the directions does not share that knowledge. She knows, in one sense, that the stranger does not know the town, else he would not be asking directions, but when she visualizes the landmarks along the route she is describing, she tends to proceed as though the one to whom she is giving directions has the same images in mind as she mentions them to him.

If people generally overproject their knowledge to others, it should be more common for writers, when writing for an audience that is less expert than they, to omit information the intended readers need for comprehension than to include information that they do not need. Erroneously assuming that people have knowledge they do not have can be hazardous in some instances: think of a person walking along a road with the setting sun at his back who assumes that because he can see an oncoming car, the driver of the car must be able to see him.

Whether overestimation or underestimation of what others know is the preferable direction in which to err is debatable; it is probably important not to be very far off in either direction. Overestimating others' knowledge can produce unrealistic expectations and lead to talking over peoples' heads; underestimating can result in talking down to people and being perceived as patronizing or condescending.

Limits of Projection

What does it mean to take the perspective of another person? As philosophers have been pointing out for centuries, there is no way that Person A can verify that the experience he has when he sees red is the same experience that Person B has when she sees red. They may look at the same color and call it by the same name, but who knows whether what they *see* is the same? Nevertheless, each of us thinks he or she can understand another's state of mind when the other says he or she is happy, sad, in pain, contented, confused, euphoric, or worried, because we know what it is to be a human being and to be happy, sad, in pain, and so on. We do not understand what it is like for a dog, a cat, or a goldfish to be happy, sad, in pain, or contented; one may even doubt that these words are descriptive of their mental states, or that such creatures even have mental states as we understand them.

What was it like to be George Washington, Mother Teresa, Babe Ruth, Joseph Stalin? We get hints of many kinds from the accounts of their lives, but our main resource is our first-hand knowledge of what it is like to be ourselves. We imagine ourselves in their times and situations, and assume that they felt the way we think we would feel.

In his story "Metamorphosis," Franz Kafka describes the reactions of Gregor Samsa, who, upon awakening one day, finds himself transformed into a "verminous bug." We can be sure that Kafka did not know what it is like to be a bug—only, perhaps, what it would be like to be a man in the body of a bug. (Perhaps not even that.) What it is like to be a bug is known only, if at all, by a bug.

• A man can understand that the experience of childbirth is profound, that it is typically attended by a mixture of severe pain and inexpressible joy, but, as a male, he cannot really know what it is like to give birth to a child.

• A sighted and hearing person cannot know what it is like to be born blind, or deaf. One can try to imagine it, but it seems safe to assume that whatever one imagines does not match the reality.

• The vast majority of us cannot know what it is like to be the president of the United States. Again, we can try to imagine it, and our imaginations get help from many sources because the president's life is much in the news. So one can be aware of many of the situations in which he finds himself, and of the ways in which he reacts to those situations. But, excepting those who have actually held the office, one cannot really know what it is like to *be* the president.

• An unschooled person from a primitive culture cannot understand how a nuclear physicist conceives the physical world; but it seems equally unlikely that the physicist can see the world through the eyes of the unschooled person from a primitive culture.

• A person who has never experienced incapacitating terror at the very thought of speaking in public may understand that stage fright can be incapacitating, but not appreciate the feeling of panic that a person who is phobic about public speaking may experience. A person who has experienced severe homesickness has no trouble empathizing with someone else who is experiencing it; people who have never been homesick may find it hard to imagine just how miserable a truly homesick person feels.

In short, when one attempts to imagine what it is like to be a specific other person, what one is really doing is imagining what it would be like to be oneself—how one would feel or behave—in the other person's situation. To feel another's pain or joy is to imagine one's own feelings if faced with whatever it is that is producing the pain or joy that the other is experiencing. One can never be certain that one's own imagined experience in the imagined situation would be, in fact, the same at that of another person who is actually in that situation. The assumption of a close correspondence seems essential to empathy, but it is also important to recognize that the assumption could be wrong in many specific instances.

Naturalness of Empathy

It seems the most natural thing in the world to attempt to put oneself—emotionally or mentally—in the place of another person, to try to imagine what the other is feeling or thinking. Not only do we often intentionally attempt to imagine what may be in another person's mind, we also impute knowledge and feelings to people without being conscious of doing so. Much of the common ground that plays a critical role in communication—whether by shaping utterances, as the audience-design hypothesis contends, or by correcting errors of comprehension, as the monitoring-and-adjustment hypothesis claims—is tacit and probably not even consciously recognized as instrumental unless brought to one's attention.

The results of many experiments, some mentioned above and others like them, support the general notion that people tend to use their own knowledge or their assumed knowledge—their model of their own knowledge—as a default indication of what other people are likely to know. From one point of view, it seems clear that this is a very sensible thing to do. If most of what most people know is "common knowledge," then, on average, when one assumes that a random other person probably has a particular bit of knowledge in common with oneself, one is more likely to be right than wrong. And the likelihood of being right undoubtedly increases to the extent that the other person is one's peer in some nontrivial sense (a member of the same culture, subculture, social group, profession).

On the other hand, it is clear too that using one's model of one's own knowledge as a basis for assuming what others are likely to know, or not know, can also yield miscalculations. The results of several experiments mentioned here invite the conclusion that people are quite likely to overestimate the extent to which what they know, or think they know, is known by others as well—which is to say that people are likely to consider their own knowledge to be more representative of the knowledge of others than it really is. If this conclusion is valid, we should expect people who know relatively much—about a specific topic or in general—to find it easy to overestimate what others know, and people who know relatively little to underestimate the knowledge that others have. Whether this is the case is a question for future research.

Acknowledgment

The work reported in this chapter was supported in part by National Science Foundation grant 0241739.

References

Ackerman, B. P., Szymanski, J., & Silver, D. (1990). Children's use of common ground in interpreting ambiguous referential utterances. *Developmental Psychology, 26,* 234–245.

Andersen, H. B., Pedersen, C. R., & Andersen, H. H. K. (2001). Using eye tracking data to indicate team situation awareness. In M. J. Smith, G. Salvendy, D. Harris, & R. J. Koubek (Eds.), *Usability evaluation and interface design: Cognitive engineering, intelligent agents and virtual reality* (pp. 1318–1322). Mahwah, NJ: Erlbaum.

Bandura, A. (1982). Self-efficacy mechanisms in human agency. *American Psychologist, 37,* 122–147.

Bennett, M., & Hibberd, M. (1986). Availability and the false consensus effect. *Journal of Social Psychology, 126,* 403–405.

Calogero, M., & Nelson, T. O. (1992). Utilization of base-rate information during feeling-of-knowing judgments. *American Journal of Psychology, 105,* 565–573.

Cannon-Bowers, J. A., Salas, E., & Converse, S. (1993). Shared mental models in expert team decision making. In N. J. Castellan, Jr. (Ed.), *Individual and group decision making: Current issues* (pp. 221–246). Hillsdale, NJ: Erlbaum.

Cattell, R. B. (1944). Projection and the design of projective tests of personality. *Character and Personality, 12,* 177–194.

Clark, H. H., & Carlson, T. B. (1981). Context for comprehension. In J. Long & A. Baddeley (Eds.), *Attention and performance IX* (pp. 313–330). Hillsdale, NJ: Erlbaum.

Clark, H. H., & Haviland, S. E. (1977). Comprehension and the given-new contract. In R. O. Freedle (Ed.), *Discourse production and comprehension.* Norwood, NJ: Ablex.

Clark, H. H., & Marshall, C. E. (1981). Definite reference and mutual knowledge. In A. K. Joshi, I. Sag, & B. Webber (Eds.), *Elements of discourse understanding* (pp. 10–63). Cambridge: Cambridge University Press.

Clark, H. H., & Murphy, G. L. (1982). Audience design in meaning and reference. In J.-F. L. Ny & W. Kintsch (Eds.), *Language and comprehension* (pp. 287–299). Amsterdam: North Holland.

Clark, H. H., Schreuder, R., & Buttrick, S. (1983). Common ground and the understanding of demonstrative reference. *Journal of Verbal Learning and Verbal Behavior, 22,* 245–258.

Collingwood, R. G. (1946). *The idea of history.* London: Oxford University Press.

Dawes, R. M. (1989). Statistical criteria for establishing a truly false consensus effect. *Journal of Experimental Social Psychology, 25,* 1–17.

Deutsch, W., & Pechmann, T. (1982). Social interaction and the development of definite descriptions. *Cognition, 11,* 159–184.

Flavell, J. H. (1977). *Cognitive development.* Englewood Cliffs, NJ: Prentice Hall.

Fussell, S. R., & Krauss, R. M. (1991). Accuracy and bias in estimates of others' knowledge. *European Journal of Social Psychology, 21,* 445–454.

Fussell, S. R., & Krauss, R. M. (1992). Coordination of knowledge in communication: Effects of speakers' assumptions about what others know. *Journal of Personality and Social Psychology, 62,* 378–391.

Gist, M. E., & Mitchell, T. E. (1992). Self-efficacy: A theoretical analysis of its determinants and malleability. *Academy of Management Review, 17,* 183–211.

Goldings, H. J. (1954). On the avowal and projection of happiness. *Journal of Personality, 23,* 30–47.

Gordon, R. (1986). Folk psychology as simulation. *Mind and Language, 1,* 158–171.

Granberg, D., & Brent, E. (1974). Dove-hawk placements in the 1968 election: Application of social judgment and balance theories. *Journal of Personality and Social Psychology, 29,* 687–695.

Granberg, D., & Brent, E. (1983). When prophecy bends: The preference-expectation link in U. S. presidential elections, 1952–1980. *Journal of Personality and Social Psychology, 45,* 477–491.

Grandy, R. (1973). Reference, meaning, and belief. *Journal of Philosophy, 70,* 439–452.

Gutwin, C., & Greenberg, S. (2002). A descriptive framework of workspace awareness for realtime groupware. *Computer Supported Cooperative Work, 11,* 411–446.

Hayes, J. R., Flower, L., Schriver, K. A., Stratman, J. F., & Carey, L. (1987). Cognitive processes in revision. In S. Rosenberg (Ed.), *Advances in applied psycholinguistics: Vol. 2. Reading, writing and language learning* (pp. 176–240). New York: Cambridge University Press.

Henle, M. (1962). The birth and death of ideas. In H. Gruber, G. Terrell, & M. Wertheimer (Eds.), *Contemporary approaches to creative thinking* (pp. 31-62). New York: Atherton.

Hoch, S. J. (1987). Perceived consensus and predictive accuracy: The pros and cons of projection. *Journal of Personality and Social Psychology, 53,* 221–234.

Hodges, S. D., & Wegner, D. M. (1997). Automatic and controlled empathy. In W. Ickes (Ed.), *Empathic accuracy* (pp. 311–339). New York: Guilford Press.

Horton, W. S., & Keysar, B. (1996). When do speakers take into account common ground? *Cognition, 59,* 91–117.

Jacoby, L. L., Bjork, R. A., & Kelley, C. M. (1994). Illusions of comprehension, competence, and remembering. In D. Druckman & R. A. Bjork (Eds.), *Learning, remembering, believing: Enhancing human performance* (pp. 57–80). Washington, DC: National Academy Press.

Jacoby, L. L., & Kelley, C. M. (1987). Unconscious influences of memory for a prior event. *Personality and Social Psychology Bulletin, 13,* 314–336.

Karniol, R. (1990). Reading people's minds: A transformation rule model for predicting others' thoughts and feelings. In L. Berkowitz (Ed.), *Advances in experimental social psychology* (Vol. 23, pp. 211-247). New York: Academic Press.

Kassin, S. M. (1979). Consensus information, prediction, and causal attribution: A review of the literature and issues. *Journal of Personality and Social Psychology, 37,* 1966–1981.

Kassin, S. M. (1981). Distortions of the process of estimating consensus from sequential events: Expectancy and order effects. *Personality and Social Psychology Bulletin, 7,* 542–546.

Katz, D., & Allport, F. (1931). *Students' attitudes.* Syracuse, NY: Craftsman Press.

Keysar, B., Barr, D. J., Balin, J. A., & Paek, T. S. (1998). Definite reference and mutual knowledge: Process models of common ground in comprehension. *Journal of Memory and Language, 39,* 1–20.

Krueger, J. (1998). On the social perception of social consensus. In M. P. Zanna (Ed.), *Advances in experimental social psychology* (Vol. 30, pp. 163–240). New York: Academic Press.

Krueger, J., & Zeiger, J. (1993). Social categorization and the truly false consensus effect. *Journal of Personality and Social Psychology, 65,* 670–680.

Mahoney, M. J. (1977). Publication prejudices: An experimental study of confirmatory bias in the peer review system. *Cognitive Therapy and Research, 1,* 161–175.

Marks, G., & Miller, N. (1987). Ten years of research on the false-consensus effect: An empirical and theoretical review. *Psychological Review, 102,* 72–90.

Mullen, B. (1983). Egocentric bias in estimates of consensus. *Journal of Social Psychology, 121,* 31–38.

Nelson, T. O., Leonesio, R. J., Landwehr, R. S., & Narens, L. (1986). A comparison of three predictors of an individual's memory performance: The individual's feeling of knowing versus the normative feeling of knowing versus base-rate item difficulty. *Journal of Experimental Psychology: Learning, Memory, and Cognition, 12,* 279–287.

Newton, L. (1990). *Overconfidence in the communication of intent: Heard and unheard melodies.* Unpublished doctoral dissertation, Department of Psychology, Stanford University, Stanford, CA.

Nickerson, R. S. (1999). How we know—and sometimes misjudge—what others know: Imputing one's own knowledge to others. *Psychological Bulletin, 125,* 737–759.

Nickerson, R. S. (2001). The projective way of knowing: A useful heuristic that sometimes misleads. *Current Directions in Psychological Research, 10,* 168–172.

Nickerson, R. S, Baddeley, A., & Freeman, B. (1987). Are people's estimates of what other people know influenced by what they themselves know? *Acta Psychologica, 64,* 245–259.

O'Mahony, J. F. (1984). Knowing others through the self: Influence of self-perception on perception of others; A review. *Current Psychological Research and Reviews, 3* (4), 48–62.

Piaget, J. (1962). Comments. Addendum to L. S. Vygotsky, *Thought and language* (E. Haufmann & G. Vakar, Eds. & Trans.). Cambridge, MA: MIT Press.

Pufall, P. B., & Shaw, R. E. (1973). Analysis of the development of children's spatial reference systems. *Cognitive Psychology, 5,* 151–175.

Ross, L., Green, D., & House, P. (1977). The "false consensus" effect: An egocentric bias in social perception and attribution processes. *Journal of Experimental Social Psychology, 13,* 279–301.

Rouse, W. B., Cannon-Bowers, J. A., & Salas, E. (1992). The role of mental models in team performance in complex systems. *IEEE Transactions on Systems, Man, and Cybernetics, 22,* 1296–1308.

Royzman, E. B., Cassidy, K. W., & Baron, J. (2003). I know you know: Epistemic egocentrism in children and adults. *Review of General Psychology, 7,* 38–65.

Stanovich, K. E., & West, R. F. (1998). Individual differences in framing and conjunction effects. *Thinking and Reasoning, 4,* 289–317.

Steedman, M. J., & Johnson-Laird, P. N. (1980). The production of sentences, utterances and speech acts: Have computers anything to say? In B. Butterworth (Ed.), *Language production: Vol. 1. Speech and talk.* London: Academic Press.

Valins, S., & Nisbett, R. E. (1972). Attribution processes in the development and treatment of emotional disorders. In E. E. Jones, D. E. Kanouse, H. H. Kelley, R. E. Nisbett, S. Valins, & B. Weiner (Eds.), *Attribution: Perceiving the causes of behavior.* Morristown, NJ.: General Learning Press.

Wallen, R. (1943). Individuals' estimates of group opinion. *Journal of Social Psychology, 17,* 269–274.

Weiner, B., Frieze, I., Kukla, A., Reed, L., Rest, S., & Rosenbaum, R. M. (1972). Perceiving the causes of success and failure. In E. E. Jones et al. (Eds.), *Attribution: Perceiving the causes of behavior.* Morristown, NJ: General Learning Press.

5 Empathic Accuracy: Its Links to Clinical, Cognitive, Developmental, Social, and Physiological Psychology

William Ickes

During the past two decades, the research on empathic accuracy has demonstrated its potential to bridge the major areas of psychology in which the study of empathy is now concentrated: clinical, cognitive, developmental, social, and physiological psychology. In this chapter, I define the construct of empathic accuracy, describe its measurement and application in three alternative research paradigms, and review some representative findings from this tradition that are relevant to the areas of clinical, cognitive, developmental, social, and physiological psychology. I conclude the chapter by suggesting some reasons that may account for the cross-area appeal and integrative potential of empathic accuracy research.

Definitions

Empathic inference is the everyday mind reading that people do whenever they attempt to infer other people's thoughts and feelings. It is a concept that other writers address under such headings as "mentalizing" or "theory of mind" (Stone, 2006; Stone & Gerans, 2006). *Empathic accuracy* is the extent to which such everyday mind reading attempts are successful (Ickes, 1997, 2003). To put it simply, empathically accurate perceivers are those who are good at "reading" other people's thoughts and feelings.

The concept of empathic accuracy can be traced back to Carl Rogers, who used the term "accurate empathy" to describe a clinician's ability to correctly infer from one moment to the next the patient's specific thoughts and feelings (Rogers, 1957). In the work that my colleagues and I have done, the term *empathic accuracy* has essentially the same meaning, referring more generally to the degree to which a perceiver is able to accurately infer the specific content of another person's successive thoughts and feelings (Ickes, 1993, 2001, 2003). This work makes no presumptions about the processes that underlie a perceiver's empathic accuracy. Instead, it uses a video-cued procedure to measure empathic accuracy directly, and then links this measure empirically to a range of process- and outcome-relevant variables in order to gain inductive insights about the nature of everyday mind reading (Ickes, 2003).

Measurement and Alternative Research Paradigms

In the empathic accuracy research paradigm, perceivers infer the thoughts or feelings of one or more target persons from a videotaped record of a social interaction in which the target(s) have participated. Immediately following these interactions, the target persons report the actual thoughts and feelings they remember having had at specific points on the videotape. The perceivers in our studies are later asked to view the videotape and, at each of the previously identified "tape stops," infer the specific thought or feeling that the target person(s) reported at that point. When all of the data for a given study are complete, trained raters then compare the content of each actual thought or feeling with the content of the corresponding inference and assign "accuracy points" that are aggregated to create an overall index of empathic accuracy (for the details of this procedure, see Ickes, 2001).

Variations of this procedure have been used in three types of studies. In studies using the *unstructured dyadic interaction paradigm*, two participants are unobtrusively videotaped while in a "waiting room" situation. Then, after having been informed about the taping and having given their consent for its further use, the participants are seated in separate cubicles where they are asked to view their own copy of the videotape and pause it at each of the points where they distinctly remember having had a particular thought or feeling. Each participant records the specific content of each thought or feeling in sentence form on the thought/feeling recording forms that are provided.

Each participant is then asked to view the videotape a second time, on this occasion for the purpose of inferring the content of the specific thoughts or feelings that his or her interaction partner has recorded. The videotape is stopped for each participant at the appropriate times by an experimenter, and the participant records an inference about each of the interaction partner's thoughts and feelings on the thought/feeling inference forms that are provided. This paradigm is useful for studying empathic accuracy in the naturally occurring interactions of pairs of individuals whose level of acquaintance can vary widely, depending on the purposes of the study: strangers, acquaintances, friends, dating partners, or couples who are married or cohabitating (see, for example, Stinson & Ickes, 1992, and Simpson, Oriña, & Ickes, 2003).

In studies using the *standard stimulus paradigm*, each participant is asked to view one or more videotapes of interactions in which he or she was not a participant. In these studies, the participants are outside observers of other people's interactions, such as the interactions between a client and a therapist, a mother and her child, or two strangers who are meeting for the first time. Once again, the participant's task is to try to infer the specific content of each of the thoughts and feelings that were previously reported by the target person(s) who appear on the tape, using the standard thought/feeling inference forms for this purpose. Because the participants in such studies always infer the thoughts and feelings of the same target person(s) (the task is the same for all of them), it is possible to compare empathic accuracy scores across participants—something that cannot be done when the unstructured dyadic interaction paradigm is used. The standard stimulus paradigm is particularly useful in studies where the focus is on individual differences in the perceivers' empathic accuracy (Marangoni et al., 1995). It can also be used to study the cross-target consistency of these individual differences when the perceivers are asked to infer the thoughts and feelings of more than one target person (Ickes, Buysse, et al., 2000).

Finally, in studies using the *standard interview paradigm*, each participant views a videotape in which a target person is asked to respond to a standard set of questions that are posed by a trained interviewer (see, for example, Dugosh, 2001). The tape is paused after each question is asked, and the participant's task at each tape stop is to try to predict what the specific content of the target person's answer will be (again, by writing it down in sentence form on the empathic inference recording forms that have been provided). This type of study is particularly useful in studying acquaintanceship effects, because it lends itself well to yoked-subjects designs in which the perceiver pairs are composed of one perceiver who knows the target person well and one perceiver who doesn't.

In all of these research paradigms, different raters assess the degree of similarity between the perceiver's empathic inferences and the corresponding thoughts or feelings that the target person actually reported. One can therefore assess the interrater reliability of the aggregated measure of empathic accuracy, which has generally been quite high. For example, in the studies that my colleagues and I have conducted, the interrater reliabilities have ranged from a low of .85 in a study in which only four raters were used to a high of .98 in two studies in which either seven or eight raters were used. Across all of the studies conducted to date, the average interrater reliability has been about .90 (Ickes, 2001).

Over the past two decades, dozens of empathic accuracy studies have been reported. Although most of the early work was conducted in my lab at the University of Texas at Arlington, empathic accuracy research is now well established in labs throughout the United States and in other countries such as Belgium, England, New Zealand, and Switzerland. Moreover, by adapting our empathic accuracy paradigms to their own areas of expertise, researchers have demonstrated the potential of empathic accuracy research to bridge the major areas of psychology in which the study of empathy is now concentrated: clinical, cognitive, developmental, social, and physiological psychology. In the following sections, I briefly review some of the more noteworthy findings in each of these areas.

Clinical Psychology

In the area of clinical psychology, researchers have explored how empathic accuracy might be enhanced in psychotherapy and have investigated its role in a number of psychological disorders.

Psychotherapy

Marangoni and her colleagues (1995) asked 80 undergraduate perceivers to attempt to infer the specific thoughts and feelings reported by each of three female clients whose interactions with the same male therapist were recorded as standard stimulus videotapes. During the middle portion of each tape, the perceivers in the *feedback condition* were given feedback about the client's actual thought or feeling immediately after making each of their empathic inferences. In contrast, the perceivers in the *no feedback condition* received no feedback of this type. The experimenters found a significant facilitative effect of the feedback training that was evident in the perceivers' subsequent empathic inferences (Marangoni et al., 1995).

Using the Marangoni study as their point of departure, Barone and his colleagues (2005) provided a similar form of feedback training to half of the graduate students who were enrolled in different sections of a clinical psychology course. The students in the feedback condition received the feedback training at different points throughout the semester, whereas those in the control (no feedback) condition did not. As in the earlier study, the students in the feedback condition subsequently displayed better empathic accuracy than the students in the control condition, although this effect was limited to inferences about feelings rather than thoughts.

Taken together, the results of both studies suggest that the use of feedback training within the standard stimulus paradigm can be an effective way to improve therapist empathy. Whether improved therapist empathy translates into better therapeutic outcomes remains to be seen, however.

Autism

Working within a "theory of mind" framework, Baron-Cohen and his colleagues (e.g., Baron-Cohen, 1995, 2003; Baron-Cohen et al., 2001), have posited a strong link between empathic accuracy and autism. They argue that severe autism can be characterized as *mind-blindness*—an inability to accurately infer, or perhaps even to recognize the existence of, other people's thoughts and feelings. More recently, Baron-Cohen (2003) has further claimed that men, on average, are more autistic-like and less empathically accurate than women.

With regard to Baron-Cohen's claim about the link between autism and empathic ability, Roeyers and colleagues (2001) conducted a study using the standard stimulus paradigm and found evidence of impaired empathic accuracy in a sample of 19 adults with Asperger syndrome. This finding was particularly impressive because the control group was composed of 19 normally developing adults who were individually matched in IQ to the Asperger syndrome adults in a yoked-subjects design.

With regard to Baron-Cohen's claim about the link between gender and empathic ability, this claim appears to stand in need of a major qualification. Curiously, it seems to have been made without regard to the relevant empathic accuracy research, which has revealed no evidence of a reliable gender difference in empathic *ability* for participants in the mostly normally developing college student samples that have been used in this research (see Ickes, Gesn, & Graham, 2000). There is no doubt, however, that when autism is profound enough to be recognized and diagnosed, its victims are much more likely to be male than female, with a sex ratio of 4 to 5 autistic men for every autistic woman (Baron-Cohen, 1995).

Borderline Personality Disorder

With regard to therapy involving patients with borderline personality disorder (BPD), the results of a study by Flury, Ickes, and Schweinle (2008) appeared, at first glance, to confirm what clinical practitioners have long suspected: that BPD patients are above average in their ability to infer other people's thoughts and feelings. In this study, same-sex dyads were created in which one of the members scored high on a measure of BPD symptomatology, whereas the other member scored low. Although the higher-scoring members were more accurate in "reading" the thoughts and feelings of the lower-scoring members than vice versa, this effect was no longer significant when the authors controlled for a corresponding difference in the inferential difficulty of the dyad members' reported thoughts and feelings.

The authors concluded from this pattern of results that people with symptoms of border-line personality disorder are not, on average, more empathically accurate than those without. They do, however, enjoy an empathic advantage over their conversation partners because their own reported thoughts and feelings are atypical and quite difficult to "read" in comparison to those reported by their non-BPD interaction partners.

The implication of this finding for therapists is that they should guard against presuming that they can accurately infer the thoughts and feelings of their BPD patients. Instead, they should assertively and continually question these patients about the contents of their thoughts and feelings, which are likely to offer repeated surprises and unexpected insights. Indeed, including atypical, hard-to-infer thoughts and feelings as one of the characteristics of BPD in future versions of the Diagnostic and Statistical Manual of Mental Disorders might help to spread the word about this newly identified aspect of BPD.

The Empathic Inaccuracy of Maritally Abusive Men

Recently, researchers have used the empathic accuracy paradigm to study the psychology of maritally abusive men. In the first of these studies, Schweinle, Ickes, and Bernstein (2002) found that men who report abusing their own female partners were more likely than non-abusive men to presume that women are harboring critical and rejecting thoughts and feelings about their male partners. Presented with the task of inferring the thoughts and feelings of the three female clients who appeared in standard stimulus videotapes, the abusive men "saw" criticism and rejection significantly more often than it actually occurred.

In a follow-up study, Schweinle and Ickes (2007) replicated the finding that maritally abusive husbands are biased to infer that women are harboring critical or rejecting thoughts and feelings about their male partners in instances when women do not actually harbor those sentiments. In addition, they found that maritally abusive husbands can sustain this biased way of perceiving women by means of two independent mechanisms: (1) emotional countercontagion in the form of contemptuous reactions to women, and (2) attentional disengagement, in which the men "tune out" women's attempts to express their actual thoughts and feelings. In essence, maritally abusive husbands have already prejudged women's thoughts and feelings to be critical and rejecting, and they behave aggressively to the extent that they can sustain this biased prejudgment through feelings of contempt or by ignoring the cues that might reveal what the woman actually thinks and feels.

In the most recent study of this series, Clements and colleagues (2007) found that violent husbands had significantly lower empathic accuracy for their wives than nonviolent and nondistressed husbands had for their wives. Other comparisons in the data showed that the level of empathic accuracy among the violent husbands was uniquely low. First, their empathic accuracy for their wives was low relative to their empathic accuracy for female strangers. Second, it was also low in comparison to the empathic accuracy that male objective observers had for the wives of these violent men. Third, it was also low relative to the empathic accuracy that the wives of these violent men displayed when inferring their husbands' thoughts and feelings. This pattern of data reveals that violent husbands have an empathic deficit that is specific to their own wives' thoughts and feelings. Like the findings of the previous two studies, these findings suggest that abusive men are motivated to *avoid* understanding their wives' thoughts and feelings as a way of maintaining control within the relationship.

Cognitive Psychology

In two conceptually similar studies, Gesn and Ickes (1999) and Hall and Schmid Mast (2007) explored the relative contributions that different information channels make to perceivers' empathic accuracy. The perceivers in both studies made inferences about the thoughts and feelings of targets who appeared in standard stimulus videotapes. The tapes were modified from one condition to the next, however, to remove a particular channel of information (e.g., the words, the paralinguistic cues, the visual information), thereby enabling the researchers to determine how much the loss of a particular information channel impaired the perceivers' empathic accuracy.

In both studies, compared to when participants viewed the original tape, (1) the loss of the verbal information (the words themselves) dramatically impaired empathic accuracy; (2) the loss of the paralinguistic cues had a more moderate effect; and (3) the loss of the visual information had a surprisingly negligible effect. These findings suggest that future research should seek to determine how perceivers infer the content of other people's thoughts and feelings from the specific words they use and the manner in which they combine and order those words in the speech acts they construct.

Developmental Psychology

Empathic accuracy has also been studied in the context of child and adolescent development, though only a couple of pioneering studies have been conducted so far.

Mothers' Empathic Accuracy and Their Children's Self-Esteem

Crosby (2002) videotaped mother-child conversations in which the mother and her child (aged 9 to 11) discussed decisions they were in the process of making, such as planning a trip, making a purchase, or choosing a pet. After obtaining the children's actual thoughts and feelings during the conversation, Crosby asked each mother to infer her child's thoughts and feelings while viewing the videotape of their discussion. She found that the mothers who were the most accurate had the children with the most positive self-concepts. Even more intriguing was Crosby's additional discovery that the empathic accuracy of mothers who had experienced separations from their child through joint custody arrangements was significantly lower than that of mothers who had not.

Crosby's findings were correlational and do not establish cause and effect. Nevertheless, they are the first to suggest that empathic accuracy plays an important role in the mother-child relationship. Although it is still too early to claim that empathically accurate mothers contribute more to their children's self-esteem than less accurate mothers do, these results suggest that they might. This pioneering study should encourage other researchers to try to replicate and further clarify the meaning of Crosby's findings.

Empathic Accuracy in the Peer Relations and Adjustment of Young Adolescents

Gleason, Jensen-Campbell, and Ickes (2007) conducted a study to determine whether the empathic accuracy of young adolescents is associated with the quality of their peer relations and with their own personal adjustment. The participants were 116 young adolescents (fifth through eighth graders). At school, they completed measures that assessed the quality of their peer relations and their personal adjustment. In the lab, their global empathic accuracy was assessed by means of a standard stimulus videotape that depicted excerpts from the interactions between other children and adult teachers. To supplement these data, the parents and teachers of our adolescent participants provided independent assessments of the children's adjustment, thereby helping to counter any bias in the children's self-reports.

The results of this study revealed several interesting findings. First, the children with lower empathic accuracy were more likely to have been the target of relational victimization by their classmates. Second, the children with lower empathic accuracy were also more likely to suffer from internalizing problems such as unhappiness and depression. Third, the negative impact of lower empathic accuracy on these internalizing problems was mitigated for children who had good-quality peer relations. Fourth, and analogously, the negative impact of poor peer relations on personal adjustment was mitigated for children who had higher empathic accuracy. Taken together, these findings reveal that empathic accuracy plays a direct as well as a moderating role in the personal and social adjustment of young adolescents.

Social Psychology

Research conducted by social psychologists has explored how empathic accuracy develops between partners, the validity of the stereotype about "women's intuition," and the ways that empathic accuracy can affect the functioning of close relationships.

The Acquaintanceship Effect

In two studies using the unstructured dyadic interaction paradigm, Stinson and Ickes (1992) and Graham (1994) found that the empathic accuracy of same-sex friends was about 50 percent greater than that of same-sex strangers—a significant difference in both investigations. The data from both studies further indicated that the friends' empathic advantage was due to their greater preexisting store of mutually shared knowledge, rather than to greater similarity in the friends' personalities or to the greater level of interactional involvement they displayed.

Complementing these findings, Marangoni et al. (1995) found that a significant "acquaintanceship effect" could develop fairly quickly in a situation in which the target persons are willing to disclose at a high level. In this study, the participants viewed videotapes of psychotherapy sessions in which three different female clients interacted with the same male therapist. When the accuracy of the empathic inferences that the participants made at the start of each therapy session was compared with the accuracy of their inferences at the end of each session, a strong overall acquaintanceship effect was obtained.

This effect was not unqualified, however. One of the three female clients had thoughts and feelings that were very difficult to "read" because of her highly ambivalent feelings about the issue she discussed with the therapist. Although the acquaintanceship effect was strongly evident for the other two clients, it was weak and nonsignificant for this ambivalent and difficult-to-read client.

Other qualifications of this effect have been reported by Gesn (1995) and by Thomas, Fletcher, and Lange (1997). Gesn (1995) found that the acquaintanceship effect depended less on the length of the partners' acquaintance per se than on the degree of closeness that developed between them during this time. And Thomas, Fletcher, and Lange (1997) reported the more surprising finding that, beginning a year or two after their marriages, the empathic accuracy of married couples does not continue to increase but instead significantly *declines*. The authors proposed that this decline occurs when the respective concerns of the husband and wife diverge to the extent that they each become preoccupied with their own concerns and find it more difficult to "stay in sync with" their partner.

Gender Differences in Empathic Accuracy: Reality or Myth?

A widely held social stereotype presumes that "women's intuition" makes them better mind readers than men, but does this stereotype reflect reality or simply promulgate a myth?

The results of a relevant meta-analytic study by Ickes, Gesn, and Graham (2000) have helped to resolve this issue. The data indicate that, in normally developing individuals, the average woman does not appear to have more empathic ability than the average man. However, when situational cues remind women that they are supposed to be the more empathic gender, women will at times outperform men on empathic accuracy tasks because of greater *motivation* to do well (and not because of greater empathic ability). Furthermore, the results of studies by Klein and Hodges (2001) suggest that even this motivation-based difference can be eliminated when experimenters sufficiently engage men's motivation by paying them to be more empathically accurate!

There are, of course, reliable gender differences in other aspects of empathic responding. With regard to empathic accuracy, however, the difference between the genders appears to be the exception rather than the rule, and to be based on motivation rather than ability.

Empathic Accuracy in Close Relationships

The role of empathic accuracy in close relationships has been a topic of major interest to researchers, generating so much research that space does not permit me to review the burgeoning literature on this topic. A good place to begin, however, is with the research relevant to the empathic accuracy model that Jeffry Simpson and I have proposed (Ickes & Simpson, 1997, 2001). The studies most relevant to this model are those reported by Ickes, Dugosh, Simpson, and Wilson (2003), Simpson, Ickes, and Blackstone (1995), Simpson, Ickes, and Grich (1999), and Simpson, Oriña, and Ickes (2003).

Physiological Psychology

In one of the first studies of its type, Levenson and Ruef (1992) asked 31 perceivers to infer the changing emotional states of a husband and a wife who appeared in two different videotaped discussions. Before viewing these discussions, each perceiver was hooked up to the same physiological recording devices that the marriage partners themselves had been hooked up to. (The output from these devices enabled the researchers to track the changes in the perceiver's own physiology that occurred while he or she was attempting to infer the successive emotional states of the designated spouse in each of two videotaped discussions.) Just as the spouses themselves had done, the perceiver used a joystick control throughout each discussion to make a continuous record of the inferred positivity or negativity of the target spouse's emotional states.

Using sophisticated statistical analyses, Levenson and Ruef were able to correlate the degree of physiological synchrony between the perceiver and the target spouse with the perceiver's level of accuracy in inferring the target spouse's changing emotional states. Their results revealed that the degree of physiological linkage was strongly related to the perceivers' accuracy in inferring the target persons' *negative* emotions, but was only weakly related to the perceivers' accuracy in inferring the target person's *positive* emotions. These findings set the stage for the recent surge of interest in linking physiological measures to measures of empathy.

On the Appeal and Integrative Potential of Empathic Accuracy Research

What accounts for the appeal and the integrative potential of empathic accuracy research across areas as diverse as clinical, cognitive, developmental, social, and physiological psychology? I suggest that there are at least four reasons: (1) the measurement of empathic accuracy as a performance variable rather than as a self-report variable; (2) the design flexibility afforded by the three research paradigms that have been developed for the study of empathic accuracy; (3) the large body of evidence supporting the reliability and validity of the empathic accuracy measure; and (4) the "theory neutral" nature of the empathic accuracy construct itself.

Performance versus Self-Report

Unlike most individual difference measures that have been applied to the study of empathy, ours is a performance-based measure. Rather than assessing people's self-reported beliefs about their empathic ability, our measure assesses how well they can actually infer the specific content of other people's thoughts and feelings. This difference is important: the available research data show that self-report measures of empathically relevant dispositions (1) generally do not correlate with our performance measure of empathic accuracy (Davis & Kraus, 1997; Ickes, 2003, chap. 7), and (2) do not appear to predict important life outcome measures as well as our empathic accuracy measure does (Gleason, Jensen-Campbell, & Ickes, 2007). Empathic accuracy research offers the advantage of capturing people's actual ability to "read" others rather than just their perceived ability to do so.

Flexibility

As we have seen, empathic accuracy data can be collected using any of three research paradigms that my colleagues and I have developed: the unstructured dyadic interaction paradigm, the standard stimulus paradigm, and the standard interview paradigm. The first of these paradigms is particularly useful in observational studies of naturally occurring interaction; the second is useful in experimental studies in which different versions of the stimulus tapes are used in the different experimental conditions; and the third is useful in studies comparing how well different perceivers can predict the target person's interview responses. Although these three paradigms will undoubtedly be complemented by others that have yet to be developed, they provide a great deal of design flexibility to researchers working in various areas of psychology.

Reliability and Validity

A large body of research evidence now attests to the reliability and validity of the empathic accuracy measure (for a review, see Ickes, 2003). Within the standard stimulus paradigm, the measure has proved to be reliable between raters, between items, and across targets (Ickes, 2001; Marangoni et al., 1995; Gesn & Ickes, 1999; Schmid Mast & Ickes, 2007). And for the body of work that extends over the various research areas discussed above, the cumulative evidence for the validity of the empathic accuracy measure is impressive. Another reason for the measure's interdisciplinary appeal, then, is the compelling evidence for its reliability and construct validity.

Theory Neutral

The broad appeal and integrative potential of empathic accuracy research also derives from the "theory neutral" nature of the empathic accuracy construct. Unlike measures of perspective taking or emotional intelligence, which require theoretical assumptions about how empathy "works" (e.g., empathy works by taking the other person's perspective; empathy works through the application of pre-specified forms of emotional intelligence), our measure makes no presumptions about the processes that underlie a perceiver's empathic accuracy. Instead, we measure empathic accuracy directly, using some variation of our video-cued procedure, and then link this measure empirically to various process and outcome variables. This research strategy enables us to gain inductive insights about the nature of everyday mind reading (Ickes, 2003).

Clearly, researchers need not make an implicit, a priori commitment to a particular process view of empathy, about which they may have their doubts. Instead of placing a specific bet that the phenomenon they are studying is driven by perspective taking, emotional intelligence, or theory of mind, for example, they can simply measure empathic accuracy and let the resulting data inform them about the processes that underlie this extraordinary ability.

Conclusion

In the roughly twenty years since the research on empathic accuracy was first introduced, the three paradigms developed by the researchers in this area have been adopted, adapted, and successfully applied by researchers in all of the major areas of psychology where the study of empathy is now concentrated: clinical, cognitive, developmental, social, and physiological psychology. Collectively, the results of this work are impressive. What accounts for the broad appeal and integrative potential of empathic accuracy research? I have proposed four reasons: (1) the measurement of empathic accuracy as a performance variable rather than as a self-report variable; (2) the design flexibility afforded by the three research paradigms that have been developed for the study of empathic accuracy; (3) the large body of evidence supporting the reliability and validity of the empathic accuracy measure; and (4) the "theory neutral" nature of the empathic accuracy construct.

References

Baron-Cohen, S. (1995). *Mindblindness: An essay on autism and theory of mind.* Cambridge, MA: MIT Press.

Baron-Cohen, S. (2003). *The essential difference: The truth about the male and female brain.* New York: Basic Books.

Baron-Cohen, S., Wheelwright, S., Skinner, R., Martin, J., & Clubley, E. (2001). The Autism-Spectrum Quotient (AQ): Evidence from Asperger syndrome/high-functioning autism, males and females, scientists and mathematicians. *Journal of Autism and Communication Disorders, 31,* 5–17.

Barone, D. F., Hutchings, P. S., Kimmel, H. J., Traub, H. L., Cooper, J. T., & Marshall, C. M. (2005). Increasing empathic accuracy through practice and feedback in a clinical interviewing course. *Journal of Social and Clinical Psychology, 24,* 156–171.

Clements, K., Holtzworth-Munroe, A., Schweinle, W., & Ickes, W. (2007). Empathic accuracy of intimate partners in violent versus nonviolent relationships. *Personal Relationships, 14,* 369–388.

Crosby, L. (2002). *The relation of maternal empathic accuracy to the development of self concept.* Unpublished doctoral thesis, Fielding Institute, Santa Barbara, CA.

Davis, M. H., & Kraus, L. (1997). Personality and empathic accuracy. In W. Ickes (Ed.), *Empathic accuracy* (pp. 144–168). New York: Guilford Press.

Dugosh, J. W. (2001). *Effects of relationship threat and ambiguity on empathic accuracy in dating couples.* Unpublished doctoral thesis, University of Texas at Arlington.

Flury, J. M., Ickes, W., & Schweinle, W. (2008). The borderline empathy effect: Do high BPD individuals have greater empathic ability? Or are they just more difficult to "read"? *Journal of Research in Personality, 42,* 312–322.

Gesn, P. R. (1995). *Shared knowledge between same-sex friends: Measurement and validation.* Unpublished master's thesis, University of Texas at Arlington.

Gesn, P. R., & Ickes, W. (1999). The development of meaning contexts for empathic accuracy: Channel and sequence effects. *Journal of Personality and Social Psychology, 77,* 746–761.

Gleason, K. A., Jensen-Campbell, L., & Ickes, W. (2007). *The role of empathic accuracy in adolescents' peer relations and adjustment.* Manuscript under editorial review.

Graham, T. (1994). *Gender, relationship, and target differences in empathic accuracy.* Unpublished master's thesis, University of Texas at Arlington.

Hall, J. A., & Schmid Mast, M. (2007). *Sources of accuracy in the empathic accuracy paradigm.* Manuscript under editorial review.

Ickes, W. (1993). Empathic accuracy. *Journal of Personality, 61,* 587–610.

Ickes, W. (2001). Measuring empathic accuracy. In J. A. Hall & F. J. Bernieri (Eds.), *Interpersonal sensitivity: Theory and measurement* (pp. 219–241). Mahwah, NJ: Erlbaum.

Ickes, W. (2003). *Everyday mind reading: Understanding what other people think and feel.* Amherst, NY: Prometheus Books.

Ickes, W. (Ed.). (1997). *Empathic accuracy.* New York: Guilford Press.

Ickes, W., Buysse, A., Pham, H., Rivers, K., Erickson, J. R., Hancock, M., Kelleher, J., & Gesn, P. R. (2000). On the difficulty of distinguishing "good" and "poor" perceivers: A social relations analysis of empathic accuracy data. *Personal Relationships, 7,* 219–234.

Ickes, W., Dugosh, J. W., Simpson, J. A., & Wilson, C. L. (2003). Suspicious minds: The motive to acquire relationship-threatening information. *Personal Relationships, 10,* 131–148.

Ickes, W., Gesn, P. R., & Graham, T. (2000). Gender differences in empathic accuracy: Differential ability or differential motivation? *Personal Relationships, 7,* 95–109.

Ickes, W., & Simpson, J. A. (1997). Managing empathic accuracy in close relationships. In W. Ickes (Ed.), *Empathic accuracy* (pp. 218–250). New York: Guilford Press.

Ickes, W., & Simpson, J. A. (2001). Motivational aspects of empathic accuracy. In G. J. O. Fletcher & M. S. Clark (Eds.), *Interpersonal processes: Blackwell handbook in social psychology* (pp. 229–249). Oxford: Blackwell.

Klein, K. J. K., & Hodges, S. (2001). Gender differences, motivation, and empathic accuracy: When it pays to understand. *Personality and Social Psychology Bulletin, 27,* 720–730.

Levenson, R. W., & Ruef, A. M. (1992). Empathy: A physiological substrate. *Journal of Personality and Social Psychology, 63,* 234–246.

Marangoni, C., Garcia, S., Ickes, W., & Teng, G. (1995). Empathic accuracy in a clinically relevant setting. *Journal of Personality and Social Psychology, 68,* 854–869.

Roeyers, H., Buysse, A., Ponnet, K., & Pichal, B. (2001). Advancing advanced mind-reading tests: Empathic accuracy in adults with a pervasive developmental disorder. *Journal of Child Psychology and Psychiatry, 42,* 271–278.

Rogers, C. R. (1957). The necessary and sufficient conditions of therapeutic personality change. *Journal of Consulting Psychology, 21,* 95–103.

Schmid Mast, M. S., & Ickes, W. (2007). Empathic accuracy: Measurement and potential clinical applications. In T. F. D. Farrow and P. W. R. Woodruff (Eds.), *Empathy and mental illness and health* (pp. 408–427). Cambridge: Cambridge University Press.

Schweinle, W. E., & Ickes, W. (2007). The role of men's critical/rejecting overattribution bias, affect, and attentional disengagement in marital aggression. *Journal of Social and Clinical Psychology, 26,* 173–198.

Schweinle, W. E., Ickes, W., & Bernstein, I. H. (2002). Empathic inaccuracy in husband to wife aggression: The overattribution bias. *Personal Relationships*, *9*, 141–158.

Simpson, J., Ickes, W., & Blackstone, T. (1995). When the head protects the heart: Empathic accuracy in dating relationships. *Journal of Personality and Social Psychology*, *69*, 629–641.

Simpson, J. A., Ickes, W., & Grich, J. (1999). When accuracy hurts: Reactions of anxious-uncertain individuals to a relationship-threatening situation. *Journal of Personality and Social Psychology*, *76*, 754–769.

Simpson, J. A., Oriña, M. M., & Ickes, W. (2003). When accuracy hurts, and when it helps: A test of the empathic accuracy model in marital interactions. *Journal of Personality and Social Psychology*, *85*, 881–893.

Stinson, L., & Ickes, W. (1992). Empathic accuracy in the interactions of male friends versus male strangers. *Journal of Personality and Social Psychology*, *62*, 787–797.

Stone, V. E. (2006). Theory of mind and the evolution of social intelligence. In J. T. Cacioppo, P. S. Visser, & C. L. Pickett (Eds.), *Social neuroscience: People thinking about thinking people* (pp. 103–129). Cambridge, MA: MIT Press.

Stone, V. E., & Gerans, P. (2006). What's domain-specific about theory of mind? *Social Neuroscience*, *1* (3–4), 309–319.

Thomas, G., Fletcher, G. J. O., & Lange, C. (1997). On-line empathic accuracy in marital interaction. *Journal of Personality and Social Psychology*, *72*, 839–850.

6   Empathic Responding: Sympathy and Personal Distress

Nancy Eisenberg and Natalie D. Eggum

Empathy appears to exist in some nonhuman species (Preston & de Waal, 2002), and evidence of empathic responding (i.e., offering help or comfort to another in distress, evidence of empathy or sympathy) has been reported or observed in children as early as the second year of life (e.g., Zahn-Waxler, Radke-Yarrow, & King, 1979; see Eisenberg, Fabes, & Spinrad, 2006). Scholars have posited various levels of human and animal empathic responding within both top-down (i.e., cognitive or attributionally driven; e.g., Hauser, 2000) and bottom-up (i.e., perceptual or sensory driven; e.g., de Waal, 2004) frameworks. The levels of empathy described often range from very rudimentary forms (e.g., emotional contagion or affective resonance) to those involving a high level of cognitive perspective taking (see Preston & de Waal, 2002).

In this chapter we discuss theory and research pertaining to the role of self-regulation—especially as reflected in effortful control—in empathy-related responding. Effortful control has been linked to neurological functioning and, hence, is relevant to the discussion of the role of the brain in empathy-related responding. In addition, work on pain and its regulation is discussed because of its theoretical association with the neurological bases of empathy. Before turning to these topics, we briefly discuss some definitional and conceptual issues.

Empathy-Related Responding

Definitions of empathy have varied considerably over the decades, from those that are cognitive in nature to those involving emotion. Eisenberg and colleagues defined *empathy* as an affective response that stems from the apprehension or comprehension of another's emotional state or condition, and which is similar to what the other person is feeling or would be expected to feel (Eisenberg et al., 1991). In Eisenberg's view, empathy requires some differentiation of one's own and the other's emotional states, as well as some level of awareness of the distinction (Eisenberg & Strayer, 1987).

Eisenberg hypothesized that empathy, if above some minimal threshold, is likely to evolve into sympathy, personal distress, or both (perhaps alternating). *Sympathy* is an emotional response, stemming from the apprehension of another's emotional state or condition, that is not the same as the other's state or condition but consists of feelings of sorrow or concern for the other (Eisenberg et al., 1991). Others have sometimes labeled sympathy as empathy or have included such responding in their definitions of empathy (e.g., Batson, 1991; Hoffman, 2000). In contrast, *personal distress* is a self-focused, aversive affective reaction to the apprehension of another's emotion, associated with the desire to alleviate one's own, but not the other's distress (e.g., discomfort, anxiety; Batson, 1991). Eisenberg et al. (1991) suggested that in addition to stemming directly from affective empathy, sympathy and personal distress may initially arise from purely cognitive processes (such as perspective taking or memory retrieval) and, in the case of personal distress, perhaps guilt. Sympathy and personal distress are hypothesized, and often found, to relate differentially to prosocial behavior (i.e., behavior intended to benefit another), and these reactions are attributed to the different motivations respectively associated with them (see Batson, 1991; Eisenberg & Fabes, 1990; Eisenberg et al., 2006).

In thinking about what determines the experience of sympathy versus personal distress, Eisenberg and Fabes (1992) suggested that empathic overarousal induced by viewing another's negative emotion promotes a self-focus—that is, personal distress—and a desire to alleviate one's own, but not the other's, negative arousal. Personal distress generally has been negatively related or unrelated to prosocial behavior when the actor can escape contact with the person evoking the distress, whereas sympathy tends to be positively related (Batson, 1991; Eisenberg et al., 2006). In contrast, optimal levels of arousal are hypothesized to promote an other-focus, and therefore are expected to be associated with sympathy and prosocial behavior. People who experience very low levels of empathy are expected to have difficulty sympathizing (and, indeed, are prone to psychopathic tendencies; see, for example, Blair, 1999). Thus, individuals most likely to experience empathy may be those prone to at least moderate levels of vicarious emotion, and among those individuals, those who are well regulated are expected to be the most sympathetic (Eisenberg et al., 1996). If an individual is prone to intense emotions, but is not well regulated, he or she is expected to be biased to experience overarousal and, therefore, personal distress. Research by Eisenberg and colleagues has generally supported these theoretical assertions (Eisenberg et al., 2006; for review see Eisenberg, Valiente, & Champion, 2004).

Eisenberg's view is highly similar to that of Decety and Jackson (2004), who argued that there are three functional components of empathy: affective sharing between the self and the other, self-other awareness, and mental flexibility and self-regulation. The first component includes shared representations between the self and others, and relies on automatic perception and action coupling or activation of emotions. Decety and Jackson suggested that the neural bases of affective sharing are widely distributed. The second component, self-other awareness, is the knowledge that self and other are similar but separate; it likely involves the right inferior parietal cortex and prefrontal areas. The third component, mental flexibility and self-regulation, assists in consciously engaging in perspective taking and maintaining conscious engagement in perspective taking and maintenance of clear self-other separation. Self-regulation allows one to inhibit one's own perspective and evaluate the perspective of another. Mental flexibility and self-regulation are believed to involve the prefrontal cortex and other areas associated with executive function and regulation of emotion. Decety and Jackson's perspective, like that of Eisenberg and her colleagues, highlights the cognitive component (i.e., the need to comprehend the other's state), the criterion of differentiating at some level between self and other, the affective component of empathy, and the importance of regulatory processes in empathy-related responding.

One way these views differ is that Eisenberg and colleagues have not emphasized the role of emotion regulation in empathy; they have argued that it is most important for sympathy, a response for which the modulation of emotional experience appears to be crucial. We heartily agree with Decety and Jackson (2004), however, that regulation of cognitive processes is essential for empathy (as it is for sympathy)—"that the mental flexibility to adopt someone else's point of view is an effortful and controlled process" (Decety & Jackson, 2004, p. 84). Moreover, Decety and Jackson apparently agree with us that the regulation of vicarious emotion also is essential; they asserted:

Empathy . . . necessitates some level of emotion regulation to manage and optimize intersubjective transactions between self and other. Indeed, the emotional state generated by the perception of the other's state or situation needs regulation and control for the experience of empathy. Without such control, the mere activation of the shared representation, including the associated autonomic and somatic responses, would lead to emotional contagion or emotional distress. (2004, p. 87)

This statement is consistent with Eisenberg's argument that regulation is essential to keep high levels of vicarious emotional arousal from turning into personal distress.

Decety and Jackson (2004), like Eisenberg, appear to differentiate between simple emotional contagion and empathy. Other researchers sometimes include emotional contagion in empathy, but may differentiate among various types of empathy. Preston and de Waal (2002) included emotional contagion in the construct of empathy and hypothesized that empathic responding may be processed via two pathways. The subcortical route is believed to be quick and reflexive and to encompass contagious forms of empathy, whereas the cortical route is likely slower and probably corresponds to cognitive forms of empathy. In our view, the first of these routes is likely to lead to emotional contagion or perhaps primitive forms of empathy involving minimal levels of self-other differentiation, whereas the second seems to reflect cognitive perspective taking but not necessarily the sharing of emotion. We believe empathy involves both an affective component and some level of cognition (see Eisenberg, 2002; also Gallese, Ferrari, & Umiltà, 2002).

Decety and Jackson (2004) provided an excellent review of the literature supporting the view that shared representations and self-other differentiation play a role in empathy. They also reviewed the neuroscience research relevant to the circuits involved, including work on mirror neurons (see Grèzes & Decety, 2001; Rizzolatti, Fogassi, & Gallese, 2001), on self-awareness (e.g., Keenan, Gallup, & Falk, 2003), and on a sense of agency (i.e., distinguishing between self-produced actions and actions generated by others; Jackson & Decety, 2004). In addition, reviews of research demonstrating that infants and children share others' emotions are readily available (see Decety & Jackson, 2004; Eisenberg et al., 2006). Decety and Jackson (2004) also reviewed research relevant to the neural correlates of experiencing vicariously induced emotion; they concluded that there is no specific cortical site for shared representations and that the pattern of activation varies according to the particular emotion, the domain of processing, and stored information. We do not review these bodies of work; rather, we focus the remainder of the chapter on regulatory processes linked to empathy-related responding.

Effortful Self-Regulatory Processes

Psychologists usually have studied the relation of emotion regulation to empathy-related responding at a behavioral or reported level. Initial findings support the view that regulatory processes, including some executive control skills, are associated with empathy and/or sympathy (which sometimes are not differentiated).

Self-regulatory processes discussed by developmental psychologists typically include the voluntary control of the allocation of attention, inhibition of behavior, activation of behavior, planning, and integration of information such that one can detect errors. There are individual differences in these capacities, and in childhood these differences are believed to stem partly from constitutionally based temperamental systems (which have a genetic basis but can be affected by environmental factors; Rothbart & Bates, 2006). In older children and adults, similar regulatory processes are part of constructs of personality such as constraint or conscientiousness. In Rothbart's model of temperament in children, self-regulation is a major dimension that serves to modulate behavioral and emotional reactivity. The self-regulatory aspect of temperament—labeled effortful control—involves executive attention and has been studied by neuroscientists such as Posner (see Posner & Rothbart, 2007).

Effortful control is defined as "the efficiency of executive attention—including the ability to inhibit a dominant response and/or to activate a subdominant response, to plan, and to detect errors" (Rothbart & Bates, 2006). Posner and Rothbart (2007) argued that it involves the anterior attention system, which is linked to the mid-prefrontal cortex, including the anterior cingulate gyrus (see Posner & Rothbart, 2000; see also Rothbart & Bates, 2006). Consistent with this view, when adults perform a behavioral task designed to activate the attention network system, the anterior cingulate gyrus is activated, as are some other areas such as the right and left frontal areas (e.g., Fan et al., 2005). Moreover, increased activation of lateral and medial prefrontal regions has been associated with adults' regulation of negative affect (Ochsner et al., 2002). Posner and Rothbart (2007) suggested that executive attention also is affected by the lateral ventral and basal ganglia structures and that dopamine is highly involved in executive processes. Performance on tasks related to executive attention has been linked to a variety of genes, especially dopamine-related genes (such as DRD4; see Fan et al., 2003).

In one of the few relevant studies with children, Davis, Bruce, and Gunnar (2002) investigated whether performance on tasks used in functional magnetic resonance imaging (fMRI) studies to examine the anterior attentional system was related to other behavioral and parent-reported measures of impulsivity, inhibitory control, and attention focusing. Their results partially supported Posner and Rothbart's assertions; six-year-olds' performance on these tasks was positively related to parent-reported inhibitory control and negatively related to parent-reported impulsivity. In addition, an index of reaction time on the neuropsychological tasks was positively related to performance on a behavioral delay-of-gratification task, whereas an index of accuracy was negatively related to externalizing behavior problems. Performance on the task also was negatively related to parent-reported surgency/extroversion (a factor of temperament reflecting impulsivity, tendency to approach, etc.).

In many other studies, behavioral measures of children's effortful control have been correlated with parents' and/or teachers' reports of children's dispositional effortful control (e.g., Eisenberg, Smith, et al., 2004; Kochanska, Murray, & Harlan, 2000). On both behavioral and reported measures, high levels of effortful control tend to predict low levels of children's negative emotionality and problem behaviors, and high levels of social competence (see Eisenberg et al., 2000; Eisenberg, Hofer, & Vaughan, 2007). For example, adults' ratings of preschool children's effortful attentional control were negatively related to dispositional negative emotionality, and to nonconstructive coping reactions to negative emotion in real-life situations (e.g., Eisenberg et al., 1993; Eisenberg, Fabes, Nyman, et al., 1994). These ratings also predicted socially competent behavior and low levels of problem behaviors years later (e.g., Eisenberg, Fabes, et al., 1997). Thus, measures of effortful control appear to tap self-regulatory processes involved in emotion regulation and have been linked in theoretically expected ways to other aspects of children's socioemotional functioning.

Effortful Control, Self-Regulation, and Empathy-Related Responding

As we have already discussed, Eisenberg and colleagues (e.g., Eisenberg, Fabes, Murphy, et al., 1994; Eisenberg et al., 1996) argued that individuals' tendencies to experience sympathy versus personal distress vary as a function of dispositional differences in individuals' abilities to regulate their emotions. Well-regulated people who have control over their ability to focus and shift attention are hypothesized to be prone to sympathy regardless of their emotional reactivity because they can modulate their negative vicarious emotion to maintain an optimal level of emotional arousal—one that has emotional force and enhances attention but is not so aversive and physiologically arousing that it promotes a self-focus. In contrast, people who are unable to regulate their emotion, especially if they are dispositionally prone to intense negative emotions, are hypothesized to be low in dispositional sympathy and prone to personal distress.

In support of Eisenberg's ideas, personal distress appears to be linked with higher levels of physiological arousal than is sympathy (for a review see Eisenberg, Valiente, & Champion, 2004; Eisenberg, Fabes, & Spinrad, 2006; see also Eisenberg et al., 1996). In addition, individual differences in children's adult-reported effortful control have been correlated with high sympathy or empathy and low personal distress (e.g., Eisenberg et al., 1996; Rothbart, Ahadi, & Hershey, 1994; Valiente et al., 2004), a finding that has been replicated in Indonesia (Eisenberg, Liew, & Pidada, 2001). In young adolescents, sympathy has been associated with personality conscientiousness (which also taps regulation; Del Barrio, Aluja, & García, 2004), constructive modes of coping (McWhirter et al., 2002), self-reported efficacy in self-regulation (e.g., resisting peer pressure to engage in high-risk behaviors, use of alcohol and drugs, theft, and other transgressive activities), and managing negative emotions (Bandura et al., 2003).

In adults, self-reported dispositional personal distress has been related to low levels of self-reported regulation and of coping skills as reported by friends. Although self-reported sympathy was unrelated to regulation in zero-order correlations, it was significantly positively related to regulation once the effects of individual differences in negative emotional intensity were controlled (Eisenberg, Fabes, Murphy, et al., 1994; see Okun, Shepard, & Eisenberg, 2000, for similar findings with older people). In another study, involving elderly participants, self-reported effortful control was positively related to sympathy and negatively related to personal distress (Eisenberg & Okun, 1996). Similarly, in a study of a community sample of adults, Spinella (2005) found that self-reported behavioral dysfunction associated with prefrontal cortex and related subcortical structures (i.e., impaired executive functioning) was inversely correlated with self-reported dispositional perspective taking and sympathy, whereas a positive relation was found between executive dysfunction and personal distress.

Thus, there appear to be relatively reliable associations between a variety of measures of effortful control and individual differences in sympathy (which likely stems from empathy). In contrast, empathic overarousal seems to be linked to high arousal and low effortful control. Given the link between effortful control and various neuropsychological measures, it is likely that neurological processes involved in self-regulation play an important role in empathy-related responding.

Developmental Issues

Researchers have found that infants possess very limited effortful control (or executive attention), but that this capacity improves somewhat in the second year and markedly in the third year of life (Kochanska, Murray, & Harlan, 2000; Rueda, Posner, & Rothbart, 2004) and continues to develop thereafter (e.g., Brocki & Bohlin, 2004). Researchers have hypothesized that immature prefrontal areas contribute to or underlie the poor inhibitory control commonly observed in infants (see Kinsbourne, 2002). Myelination of the prefrontal cortex, which is instrumental in inhibiting imitation and other behaviors, continues until adolescence (Fuster, 1997). In addition, children's understanding of emotions and of others' internal cognitions and feelings changes dramatically across childhood (Eisenberg, Murphy, & Shepard, 1997; Harris, 2006). Given the changes in these capacities across childhood and adolescence, it is likely that some of the neural correlates of empathy that can be imaged change with age; for example, different parts of the brain may be differentially involved in empathy at different ages. There is evidence that the neural correlates of performance on an inhibitory control task differ for six-year-olds and adults (Davis et al., 2003). Thus, not only may there be less neural activity related to the regulation of cognition and emotion in younger individuals, but the neural pattern itself may differ. In the future, it would be useful to examine neural functioning on empathy-related tasks for individuals who differ in both the cognitive components of empathy (understanding of emotions and the situations they occur in, perspective taking) and in its affective components.

Pain, Empathy, Regulation, and Attachment

Empathy for pain has been a popular topic of study within the perception-action framework, which posits that one's own neural substrates are activated by the perception of another's movements or observed experiences, and may have implications for the study of the development of empathy. Botvinick and colleagues (2005), for example, examined areas of the brain engaged in viewing facial expressions of pain and in the experience of pain in a sample of women via fMRI. They found that some of the brain areas involved with directly experiencing pain overlapped with areas involved when viewing facial expressions of pain (specifically, the dorsal anterior cingulate cortex and bilateral insulae), and that these areas also appear to be involved in processing other somatic and affective states. Botvinick and colleagues noted that the amygdala and orbitofrontal cortex were engaged when viewing facial expressions of pain, but not when directly experiencing pain. They concluded that pain and the viewing of pain expressions activate intersecting, but not identical, areas of the brain (Botvinick et al., 2005). Other researchers have found activation in the anterior cingulate cortex and anterior insula in response to felt and observed pain and have interpreted the activation as reflecting motivational, rather than sensory, properties of the painful stimulus (e.g., Jackson, Meltzoff, & Decety, 2005; also see Singer & Frith, 2005).

However, Avenanti and colleagues (2005) found a reduction in motor excitability of particular muscles in response to viewing delivery of pain to a model in the same muscle— a "mirror-matching" link between the visual representation of pain experienced by another and a somatomotor representation of feeling the same thing. They suggested that empathy for pain may involve both affective and sensorimotor components, and that empathy may be thought of as having two forms. The simple form may consist of somatic resonance (i.e., mapping external stimuli onto your own body), whereas the more complex form may consist of affective resonance. The authors further proposed that these two forms likely occur in different nodes of the neural network (Avenanti et al., 2005).

Tucker, Luu, and Derryberry (2005) made some intriguing suggestions regarding the role of regulation of pain in the development of empathy. Noting that the pain pathway extends to the cortex, including the anterior cingulate cortex and the orbitofrontal cortex, they argued that the "evaluative mechanisms engaged in many complex forms of self-regulation are extensions of mechanisms that evolved for evaluating and responding to pain" (p. 702). They further suggested that animals develop a tolerance for frustration (a response mediated by the neural systems that respond to pain), and that the elementary motive and self-regulatory processes involved may explain the involvement of the anterior cingulate cortex and insula in the emotional evaluation of events, the monitoring of conflict, and the use of effortful control. Specifically, through encephalization (a construct that explains how primitive neural structures are elaborated as more recently evolved additions modify the function of older structures), the pain system forms the foundation for learning and for the regulation of actions in context.

Tucker, Luu, and Derryberry (2005) noted that vocalization and pain overlap closely in their cerebral representation and suggested that the role of the anterior cingulate cortex in both pain evaluation and vocalization "exemplifies how the encephalization of the pain system relates to attachment, sympathy, and the development of empathy" (p. 704). Tucker and colleagues discussed what they labeled as sympathic resonance, which is an emotional response to the emotional display of another that ranges from contagion to more complex forms when intersubjective reasoning (cognitive) comes into play. They argued that emotional contagion, which shares neural substrates with the pain system, may provide the foundation for learning the association between another's pain-related vocalizations and the concept of pain or danger, and that with further encephalization, brain mechanisms related to parenting behaviors developed, allowing the recognition of pain vocalization as an expression of another's pain. In addition, they suggested that caring for another's welfare (sympathy) may stem from emotional contagion. The authors further proposed that empathy involves sophisticated operations of intelligence, including more deliberate processes of reasoning to integrate visceral emotional contagion and somatic sensorimotor mirroring, and to experience more complex forms of sympathic resonance. Intersubjective reasoning (cognitive processes through which the person is able to infer the perspective, intention, and subjective state of another) is, in their view, also required for people to experience more complex forms of vicarious responding (i.e., empathy).

The model proposed by Tucker and colleagues provides a way to link attachment processes and regulation to one another and to empathy. Attachment figures help infants to manage negative emotion and frustration and, consequently, promote the development of self-regulatory processes that may contribute to empathy and sympathy:

From a stable attachment relationship, the child develops self-regulatory operations that are not only associated with opiate release during reunion and affection, but extended intervals of psychological pain when the love relationship is frustrated. . . . Children whose early relationships do not provide for strong bonding experiences may not have the self-regulatory experience to tolerate frustration of sympathic pain in later relationships. (Tucker, Luu, & Derryberry, 2005, p. 211)

The authors proposed that sensitive parenting also fosters the development of children's shared mental representations and hence an understanding of others' internal states.

In fact, a secure attachment and sensitive, supportive parenting have been associated with children's higher levels of self-regulation (see Eisenberg, Smith, et al., 2004), understanding of others' emotions and internal states (e.g., see Thompson, 2006), and empathy/sympathy (see Eisenberg et al., 2006). In addition, there is preliminary evidence that individual differences in the capacity for effortful control mediate the relation between the quality of parenting and children's sympathetic tendencies (Eisenberg, Liew, & Pidada, 2001). Thus, the neural processes that evolved from the pain system and are linked to the parts of the brain involved in self-regulation may be critical to understanding empathy and its development.

Conclusion

It appears that neurologically based self-regulatory processes play an important role in empathy-related responding. Moreover, the evolution of the brain may explain links among empathy and attachment systems. In the future, researchers would benefit from examining the neurological correlates of experiencing sympathy and personal distress. In addition, it will be useful to map developmental changes in effortful control to changes in empathy-related responding. Finally, research that examines how effortful control and its neurological bases mediate the relation between socialization variables (e.g., attachment) and empathy-related responding could be used to test hypotheses about the effects of environmental factors such as parenting and education on the ability of people to respond with empathy.

References

Avenanti, A., Bueti, D., Galati, G., & Aglioti, S. M. (2005). Transcranial magnetic stimulation highlights the sensorimotor side of empathy for pain. *Nature Neuroscience, 8*, 955–960.

Bandura, A., Caprara, G. V., Barbaranelli, C., Gerbino, M., & Pastorelli, C. (2003). Role of affective self-regulatory efficacy in diverse spheres of psychosocial functioning. *Child Development, 74*, 769–782.

Batson, C. D. (1991). *The altruism question: Toward a social psychological answer.* Hillsdale, NJ: Erlbaum.

Blair, R. J. R. (1999). Responsiveness to distress cues in the child with psychopathic tendencies. *Personality and Individual Differences, 27*, 135–145.

Botvinick, M., Jha, A. P., Bylsma, L. M., Fabian, S. A., Solomon, P. E., & Prkachin, K. M. (2005). Viewing facial expressions of pain engages cortical areas involved in the direct experience of pain. *NeuroImage, 25*, 312–319.

Brocki, K. C., & Bohlin, G. (2004). Executive functions in children aged 6 to 12: A dimensional and developmental study. *Developmental Neuropsychology*, *26*, 571–593.

Davis, E. P., Bruce, J., & Gunnar, M. R. (2002). The anterior attention network: Associations with temperament and neuroendocrine activity in 6-year-old children. *Developmental Psychobiology*, *40*, 43–56.

Davis, E. P., Bruce, J., Snyder, K., & Nelson, C. A. (2003). The X-trials: Neural correlates of an inhibitory control task in children and adults. *Journal of Cognitive Neuroscience*, *15*, 432–443.

Decety, J., & Jackson, P. L. (2004). The functional architecture of human empathy. *Behavioral and Cognitive Neuroscience Reviews*, *3*, 71–100.

Del Barrio, V., Aluja, A., & García, L. F. (2004). Relationship between empathy and the Big Five personality traits in a sample of Spanish adolescents. *Social Behavior and Personality*, *32*, 677–682.

De Waal, F. B. M. (2004). On the possibility of animal empathy. In A. S. R. Manstead, N. Frijda, & A. Fischer (Eds.), *Feelings and emotions: The Amsterdam symposium* (pp. 381–401). Cambridge: Cambridge University Press.

Eisenberg, N. (2002). Distinctions among various modes of empathy-related reactions: A matter of importance to human relations. *Behavioral and Brain Sciences*, *25*, 33–34.

Eisenberg, N., & Fabes, R. A. (1990). Empathy: Conceptualization, measurement, and relation to prosocial behavior. *Motivation and Emotion*, *14*, 131–149.

Eisenberg, N., & Fabes, R. A. (1992). Emotion regulation and the development of social competence. In M. S. Clark (Ed.), *Review of personality and social psychology: Vol. 14. Emotion and social behavior* (pp. 119–150). Newbury Park, CA: Sage.

Eisenberg, N., Fabes, R. A., Bernzweig, J., Karbon, M., Poulin, R., & Hanish, L. (1993). The relations of emotionality and regulation to preschoolers' social skills and sociometric status. *Child Development*, *64*, 1418–1438.

Eisenberg, N., Fabes, R. A., Guthrie, I. K., & Reiser, M. (2000). Dispositional emotionality and regulation: Their role in predicting quality of social functioning. *Journal of Personality and Social Psychology*, *78*, 136–157.

Eisenberg, N., Fabes, R. A., Murphy, B., Karbon, M., Maszk, P., Smith, M., O'Boyle, C., & Suh, K. (1994). The relations of emotionality and regulation to dispositional and situational empathy-related responding. *Journal of Personality and Social Psychology*, *66*, 776–797.

Eisenberg, N., Fabes, R. A., Murphy, B., Karbon, M., Smith, M., & Maszk, P. (1996). The relations of children's dispositional empathy-related responding to their emotionality, regulation, and social functioning. *Developmental Psychology*, *32*, 195–209.

Eisenberg, N., Fabes, R. A., Nyman, M., Bernzweig, J., & Pinulas, A. (1994). The relations of emotionality and regulation to children's anger-related reactions. *Child Development*, *65*, 109–128.

Eisenberg, N., Fabes, R. A., Shepard, S. A., Murphy, B. C., Guthrie, I. K., Jones, S., Friedman, J., Poulin, R., & Maszk, P. (1997). Contemporaneous and longitudinal prediction of children's social functioning from regulation and emotionality. *Child Development*, 68, 642–664.

Eisenberg, N., Fabes, R. A., & Spinrad, T. L. (2006). Prosocial development. In N. Eisenberg (Vol. Ed.) and W. Damon & R. M. Lerner (Series Eds.), *Handbook of child psychology: Vol. 3. Social, emotional, personality development* (6th ed., pp. 646–718). Hoboken, NJ: Wiley.

Eisenberg, N., Hofer, C., & Vaughan, J. (2007). Effortful control and its socioemotional consequences. In J. J. Gross (Ed.), *Handbook of emotion regulation*. New York: Guilford Press.

Eisenberg, N., Liew, J., & Pidada, S. (2001). The relations of parental emotional expressivity with the quality of Indonesian children's social functioning. *Emotion*, 1, 107–115.

Eisenberg, N., Murphy, B., & Shepard, S. (1997). The development of empathic accuracy. In W. Ickes (Ed.), *Empathic accuracy* (pp. 73–116). New York: Guilford Press.

Eisenberg, N., & Okun, M. (1996). The relations of dispositional regulation and emotionality to elders' empathy-related responding and affect while volunteering. *Journal of Personality*, 64, 157–183.

Eisenberg, N., Shea, C. L., Carlo, G., & Knight, G. P. (1991). Empathy-related responding and cognition: A "chicken and the egg" dilemma. In W. M. Kurtines (Ed.), *Handbook of moral behavior and development: Vol. 2. Research* (pp. 63–88). Hillsdale, NJ: Erlbaum.

Eisenberg, N., Smith, C. L., Sadovsky, A., & Spinrad, T. L. (2004). Effortful control: Relations with emotion regulation, adjustment, and socialization in childhood. In R. F. Baumeister & K. D. Vohs (Eds.), *Handbook of self-regulation: Research, theory, and applications* (pp. 259–282). New York: Guilford Press.

Eisenberg, N., & Strayer, J. (1987). Critical issues in the study of empathy. In N. Eisenberg & J. Strayer (Eds.), *Empathy and its development* (pp. 3–31). Cambridge: Cambridge University Press.

Eisenberg, N., Valiente, C., & Champion, C. (2004). Empathy-related responding: Moral, social, and socialization correlates. In A. G. Miller (Ed.), *The social psychology of good and evil: Understanding our capacity for kindness and cruelty* (pp. 386–415). New York: Guilford Press.

Fan, J., Fossella, J., Sommer, T., Wu, Y., & Posner, M. I. (2003). Mapping the genetic variation of executive attention onto brain activity. *Proceedings of the National Academy of Science*, 100, 7406–7411.

Fan, J., McCandliss, B. D., Fossella, J., Flombaum, J. I., & Posner, M. I. (2005). The activation of attentional networks. *NeuroImage*, 26, 471–479.

Fuster, J. M. (1997). *The prefrontal cortex*. Philadelphia: Lippincott, Raven.

Gallese, V., Ferrari, P. F., & Umiltà, M. A. (2002). The mirror matching system: A shared manifold for intersubjectivity. *Behavioral and Brain Sciences*, 25, 35–36.

Grèzes, J., & Decety, J. (2001). Functional anatomy of execution, mental simulation, observation, and verb generation of actions: A meta-analysis. *Human Brain Mapping*, 12, 1–19.

Harris, P. L. (2006). Social cognition. In D. Kuhn & R. S. Siegler (Vol. Eds.) and W. Damon & R. M. Lerner (Series Eds.), *Handbook of child psychology: Vol. 2. Cognition, perception, and language* (6th ed., pp. 811–858). Hoboken, NJ: Wiley.

Hauser, M. D. (2000). *Wild minds: What animals really think.* New York: Holt.

Hoffman, M. L. (2000). *Empathy and moral development: Implications for caring and justice.* New York: Cambridge University Press.

Jackson, P. L., & Decety, J. (2004). Motor cognition: A new paradigm to study self-other interactions. *Current Opinion in Neurobiology, 14,* 259–263.

Jackson, P. L., Meltzoff, A. N., & Decety, J. (2005). How do we perceive the pain of others? A window into the neural processes involved in empathy. *NeuroImage, 24,* 771–779.

Keenan, J. P., Gallup, G. C., & Falk, D. (2003). *The face in the mirror: The search for the origins of consciousness.* New York: HarperCollins.

Kinsbourne, M. (2002). The role of imitation in body ownership and mental growth. In A. N. Meltzoff & W. Prinz (Eds.), *The imitative mind: Development, evolution, and brain bases* (pp. 311–330). New York: Cambridge University Press.

Kochanska, G., Murray, K. T., & Harlan, E. T. (2000). Effortful control in early childhood: Continuity and change, antecedents, and implications for social development. *Developmental Psychology, 36,* 220–232.

McWhirter, B. T., Besett-Alesch, T. M., Horibata, J., & Gat, I. (2002). Loneliness in high risk adolescents: The role of coping, self-esteem, and empathy. *Journal of Youth Studies, 5,* 69–84.

Ochsner, K. N., Bunge, S. A., Gross, J. J., & Gabrieli, J. D. E. (2002). Rethinking feelings: An fMRI study of the cognitive regulation of emotion. *Journal of Cognitive Neuroscience, 14,* 1215–1229.

Okun, M. A., Shepard, S. A., & Eisenberg, N. (2000). The relations of emotionality and regulation to dispositional empathy-related responding among volunteers-in-training. *Personality and Individual Differences, 28,* 367–382.

Posner, M. I., & Rothbart, M. K. (2000). Developing mechanisms of self-regulation. *Development and Psychopathology, 12,* 427–441.

Posner, M. I., & Rothbart, M. K. (2007). *Educating the human brain.* Washington, DC: American Psychological Association.

Preston, S. D., & de Waal, F. B. M. (2002). The communication of emotions and the possibility of empathy in animals. In S. G. Post, L. G. Underwood, J. P. Schloss, & W. B. Hurlbut (Eds.), *Altruism and altruistic love: Science, philosophy, and religion in dialogue* (pp. 284–308). New York: Oxford University Press.

Rizzolatti, G., Fogassi, L., & Gallese, V. (2001). Neurophysiological mechanisms underlying the understanding and imitation of action. *Nature Reviews Neuroscience, 2,* 661–670.

Rothbart, M. K., Ahadi, S. A., & Hershey, K. L. (1994). Temperament and social behavior in childhood. *Merrill-Palmer Quarterly*, *40*, 21–39.

Rothbart, M. K., & Bates, J. E. (2006). Temperament. In W. Damon & R. M. Lerner (Eds.), *Handbook of child psychology: Vol. 3. Social, emotional, and personality development* (6th ed., pp. 99–166). Hoboken, NJ: Wiley.

Rueda, M. R., Posner, M. I., & Rothbart, M. K. (2004). Attentional control and self-regulation. In R. F. Baumeister & K. D. Vohs (Eds.), *Handbook of self-regulation: Research, theory, and applications* (pp. 283–300). New York: Guilford Press.

Singer, T., & Frith, C. (2005). The painful side of empathy: Comment. *Nature Neuroscience*, *8*, 845–846.

Spinella, M. (2005). Prefrontal substrates of empathy: Psychometric evidence in a community sample. *Biological Psychology*, *70*, 175–181.

Thompson, R. A. (2006). The development of the person: Social understanding, relationships, conscience, self. In W. Damon & R. M. Lerner (Eds.), *Handbook of child psychology: Vol. 3. Social, emotional, and personality development* (6th ed., pp. 24–98). Hoboken, NJ: Wiley.

Tucker, D. M., Luu, P., & Derryberry, D. (2005). Love hurts: The evolution of empathic concern through the encephalization of nociceptive capacity. *Development and Psychopathology*, *17*, 699–713.

Valiente, C., Eisenberg, N., Fabes, R. A., Shepard, S. A., Cumberland, A., & Losoya, S. H. (2004). Prediction of children's empathy-related responding from their effortful control and parents' expressivity. *Developmental Psychology*, *40*, 911–926.

Zahn-Waxler, C., Radke-Yarrow, M., & King, R. A. (1979). Child-rearing and children's prosocial initiations toward victims of distress. *Child Development*, *50*, 319–330.

7 Empathy and Education

Norma Deitch Feshbach and Seymour Feshbach

Empathy is an attribute of children that has proven to be highly relevant to the educational process and educational outcomes. The interest of educators in empathy has historically centered on teacher empathy. Our own research has been in the area of student empathy, the primary focus of this chapter. We also take note of research on teacher empathy.

The work on teacher empathy has reflected the influence of Carl Rogers's approach to the therapeutic process (Carkhuff & Berenson, 1967). In the educational sphere, the teacher is analogous to the counselor or therapist and the student is analogous to the client. The assumption underlying the emphasis on teacher empathy is that empathic communication by the teacher will result in students experiencing greater understanding and acceptance, and that they will thus develop more positive attitudes toward themselves and toward schooling.

In contrast, recent interest in the relevance of empathy to education has shifted to the student learner and to the educational process. This research addresses the relationship of empathic qualities on the part of students to student social behaviors and to their academic achievement. The potential contribution of instructional modifications based on principles derived from an empathy approach has also been addressed in recent research.

Contemporary approaches conceive of empathy as a social interaction between any two individuals wherein one individual experiences the feelings of a second individual. This shared affect, while reflecting some degree of correspondence between the affect of the observer and that of the observed, is not identical. The process of empathy is currently acknowledged to be contingent on both cognitive and affective factors, the particular influence varying with the age and other attributes of the individual and with the situational context. The model proposed by Feshbach (1975, 1978) emphasizes the cognitive ability to discriminate affective states in others, the more mature cognitive ability to assume the perspective and role of another person, and the affective ability to experience emotions in an appropriate manner. Hoffman's developmental model also has three components—cognitive, affective and motivational—and focuses on empathic responsiveness to distress in others as the motivation for altruistic behavior (Hoffman, 1982, 1983).

Functions of Empathy

Study of empathy's functions has been beset with definitional concerns, methodological problems, and theoretical controversies. Nonetheless, the role of empathy as an important variable—meriting consideration and empirical study for many disciplines and most especially the field of education—has been established, and a wide array of functions have been attributed to the empathy process.

The scope of functions that empathy in children can mediate include social understanding, emotional competence, prosocial and moral behavior, compassion and caring, and regulation of aggression and other antisocial behaviors. It should be emphasized that empathy is not equivalent to these personal and interpersonal competencies, nor is it a magic elixir that automatically produces social competence and prosocial behavior. However, it is a very important factor in the matrix of developmental variables that mediate these cognitive and affective behaviors, all of which are important to schooling.

Prosocial Behaviors

The role that empathy plays in mediating prosocial and behavior has been a major interest of investigators concerned with the functions of empathy. Studies relating empathy to such prosocial behaviors as cooperation, sharing, donating, and other altruistic acts have generally yielded positive findings, especially in adults (Batson, 1991). Although investigators have found the link between empathy and prosocial behavior to be positive (Findlay, Girardi, & Coplan, 2006; Warden & Mackinnon, 2003; Zahn-Waxler et al., 1992), the association between empathy and prosocial behavior in children may vary with the empathy measure, the specific prosocial behavior studied, the age of the sample, and the situation itself (Eisenberg & Miller, 1987; Feshbach, 1998). Investigations that have addressed the relationship in children between empathy and cooperation and studies entailing the training of empathy have yielded more consistent positive outcomes (Feshbach et al., 1984).

Aggression

An inverse relationship between empathy and aggression tends to be supported by research findings, especially for males (S. Feshbach & N. D. Feshbach, 1969; N. D. Feshbach & S. Feshbach, 1982, 1998; Björkqvist, Österman, & Kaukiainen, 2000; Miller & Eisenberg, 1988). The findings for younger children are mixed, while those for older elementary-school-age children and adolescents are more consistent (Lovett & Sheffield, 2007).

The three-component cognitive-affective model of empathy suggests several mechanisms that should result in lower aggression and greater prosocial behavior in the empathic child relative to the less empathic child. The ability to discriminate and label the feelings of others is a prerequisite to taking into account others' needs when responding to social conflicts. The more advanced cognitive skill entailed in examining a conflict situation from the perspective of another person should result in a lessening of conflict.

The third component of empathy, affective responsiveness, has a special relationship to the regulation of aggression. Aggression implies the infliction of injury that may cause pain and distress. The observation of pain and distress should elicit distress in an empathic observer, even if the observer is the cause of the aggression. The inhibitory effect of empathy applies to instrumental as well as anger mediated aggressive behavior. One source of the difference between the relation of empathy to prosocial behaviors and its relation to aggressive behavior is the nature of the mediating process. Empathy may affect aggression through inhibition. No other response is required. However, for prosocial behavior to occur when the child is empathic, the prosocial response must be in the child's repertoire and must occur in the situation. Thus, if empathy training is to foster prosocial responses, it should be accompanied by specific prosocial behavioral training.

Social Prejudice

One would expect racial and ethnic prejudice—attitudes that are adverse to educational goals, to be affected by empathy. The empathic individual is more likely to understand and appreciate the perspective and feelings of members of diverse ethnic groups. Greater understanding and sharing of the feelings of the "other" should result in less prejudice, less conflict, and more positive social overtures. In a study by Doyle and Aboud (1995), children who improved the most in role-taking, a component of empathy, displayed the greatest reductions in social prejudice. Stephan and Finley (1999) noted that empathy figures directly or indirectly in the reduction of social conflict and related social prejudice through such diverse approaches as the "jigsaw classroom"(where students with different relevant information cooperate in order to solve a problem) and conflict-resolution workshops.

Academic Achievement and Emotional Intelligence

The functions of empathy in prosocial behavior, aggression, and social tolerance are relevant for social behaviors that schools seek to foster. These character-related behaviors, while important goals to educators in their own right, are also factors that indirectly influence classroom learning. However, a growing body of literature documents a more direct effect of empathy on academic achievement. Learning, particularly in the curriculum areas of reading, literature, and social studies, should be facilitated by empathy because the empathic child is better able to place him- or herself in the role of central characters portrayed in the fictional and historical readings. In addition to being better able to understand the roles and perspectives of these fictional and historical characters, the empathic child is better able to share and experience, to some degree, their feelings. These shared feelings may serve to underline and reinforce what they have read and been taught, resulting in better recall. Also, a number of educators have suggested that there is a reciprocal relationship between the process of reading and empathy, such that reading helps heighten and reinforce empathy (Budin, 2001; Cress & Holm, 2000).

In a short-term longitudinal study investigating the relationship between affective processes and academic achievement, a positive relationship was found between girls' empathy at age 8 and 9 and their reading and spelling skills at 10 and 11 years old. These relationships obtained even when initial performance on these achievement test measures was controlled (Feshbach & Feshbach, 1987). In a study of secondary school students, a positive relationship between empathy indicators and grade point average was observed (Bonner & Aspy, 1984). Also, schools in which students were involved in programs designed to increase empathy and create "caring communities" have been found to have higher scores than comparison schools on measures of higher-order reading comprehension (Kohn, 1991). These correlations reflecting a positive relationship between empathy and school achievement are supported by the findings of two experimental studies in which empathy training resulted in heightened achievement (Feshbach et al., 1984; Feshbach & Konrad, 2001).

Empathy has also been conceptualized as one of the key constituents of emotional or social intelligence (Salovey & Gruel, 2005). Emotional and social intelligence are generally viewed as contributing to individuals' effectiveness in social and work situations rather than to their cognitive achievements (Zeidner, Roberts, & Mathews, 2002). Although there is an overlap between empathy and the constructs of emotional and social intelligence, the latter focus on the effective use of emotional knowledge and on social skills and social competence, and should be distinguished from empathy.

Training for Empathy in Teachers

As noted earlier, most of the work on teacher empathy has primarily been guided by the Rogerian model of client-centered therapy and human development and growth. Central to this model of empathy are two elements: (1) the ability to understand and identify another's feelings and perspective; and (2) the ability to communicate that understanding to the individual with whom one is empathizing. The approach to teacher empathy differs from the work on children's and students' empathy in its emphasis on the critical role of communication in teacher empathy. Understanding of the student is necessary but not sufficient. The crux of teacher empathy lies in the interaction of the teacher with the student. Through teachers communicating to students their understanding of how the students feel, the latter are presumed to experience greater acceptance. Just as clients develop attachments to their counselor and to the therapeutic situation, it is believed that students who experience empathic communications from their teacher will develop attachments to the teacher and to schooling (Carkhuff & Berenson, 1967). As clients develop greater self-acceptance in response to the therapeutic experience, so should the self-esteem of students increase in response to an empathic teacher.

The results of a number of correlational studies are consistent with these theoretical expectations. Positive relationships between teacher empathy and indices of academic achievement have been found for samples of third graders (Aspy, 1971) and of college students (Chang, Berger, & Chang, 1981). There is also evidence that teacher empathy may have a positive influence on student attitudes: teacher empathy toward withdrawn students is correlated with middle-school peers' acceptance of withdrawn students in their classes (Chang, 2003).

Most of the literature on teacher empathy focuses on the investigation of ways to enhance teacher empathy. A variety of techniques, ranging from human relations training (Higgins, Moracco, & Danford, 1981) and interpersonal communication skills development (Warner, 1984), to role-playing (Kelly, Reavis, & Latham, 1977), to discussion of moral dilemmas (Black & Phillips, 1982), to lectures and programmed materials on active listening and identifying feelings (Kremer & Dietzen, 1991), have been found to be effective in enhancing teacher and teacher trainee empathy. The teacher education literature has also addressed the importance of teacher empathy in the instruction of ethnically diverse student populations (Redman, 1977).

Many of the instructional programs entail complex, multifaceted methods with varied effects, making it difficult to link a particular training component to the enhancement of empathy. A major need is for studies linking the experimental enhancement of teacher empathy to classroom student behaviors and achievement. One example is Harbach and Asbury's (1976) finding that the training of teachers in human relations and social understanding resulted in less negative classroom student behavior. Also germane is a study by Sinclair & Fraser (2002) in which they found an improvement in the classroom environment of teachers who had participated in training that had a component aimed at enhancing empathy. Experimental studies focusing directly on empathy are needed to buttress the correlational findings of relationships between teacher empathy and student performance.

Fostering Empathy among Students

Although the ontogenetic pattern of empathic development is unresolved, it is now generally accepted that empathy can be learned and therefore that empathy can be taught and trained. The programs and research dealing with empathy training in some form include diverse populations varying in sex and racial, ethnic, and cultural backgrounds. A wide age range is also represented, extending from preschoolers and elementary students to high school and college age students.

Approaches

The research can be grouped into two principal categories. One set of studies or programs focuses on methods or techniques to increase empathy, with the implication that empathy, once enhanced, will have positive consequences for growth and learning. A second group of programs, while also directly training for empathy, is oriented toward its educational consequences in the cognitive, affective, behavioral, or academic realms.

In addition to these more systematic approaches, one finds other, more informal references in magazine articles and newspapers to the use of empathy-stimulating experiences in the classroom: students being exposed to peers from different socioeconomic backgrounds, learning about poverty, learning about the Holocaust, visiting hospitals, spending time in homeless shelters, and participating in activities that aid disadvantaged groups. Unfortunately, it is difficult to ascertain specific outcomes of these presumably empathy-enhancing activities or the precise student population involved. Also, one finds in the literature a number of papers recommending (without offering any evaluations) the use of literature (Budin, 2001) or art (Stout, 1999) or history (Davis, Yeager, & Foster, 2001) as tools to stimulate empathy.

With regard to the first group of studies, which use a variety of procedures to foster empathy, evidence is accumulating that when students both young and old learn about empathy and are trained to recognize emotional states in themselves and others, their empathic skills increase (Kremer & Dietzen, 1991). Moreover, a number of studies indicate that when similarity between oneself and others is stressed, an increase in empathy occurs (Brehm, Fletcher, & West, 1981) Role taking or role playing, an activity in which the person assumes the role of a real, fictional, or historical figure, is a longtime educational strategy that appears to be highly effective in increasing both affective and cognitive empathy (Barak, Engle, Katzir, & Fisher., 1987; Feshbach, Feshbach, Fauvre, & Ballard-Campbell., 1984; Underwood & Moore, 1982). Also, training in perspective taking, the ability to take another person's point of view, another traditional educational strategy, increases levels of empathy (Feshbach et al., 1984; Feshbach & Konrad, 2001; Pecukonis, 1990). The content of the materials that are used in training is also a factor, both children and adults being especially responsive and empathic to dysphoric content. Apparently, observing misfortune inspires empathy (Barnett et al., 1982; Perry, Bussey, & Freiberg, 1981). Modeling the behavior of others, an important mechanism in learning, is another factor that influences the development of empathy (Kohn, 1991; Kremer, & Dietzen, 1991).

Interestingly, music education training also inspires empathic responding. Finnish daycare attendees who participated in a 12-hour program that included a variety of musical activities—singing, playing instruments, listening to music and to lyrics dealing with empathy and prosocial behavior—manifested an increase in empathy and prosocial behavior (Hietolahti-Ansten & Kalliopuska, 1991; Kalliopuska & Ruokonen, 1993). Cross-age tutoring is another educational strategy to stimulate the development of empathy, as are the many variations of cooperative learning (Aronson & Patnoe, 1997; Yogev & Ronen, 1982). Cooperative learning curriculum involves group learning and mutual dependence, and is believed by Aronson and Patnoe to improve student achievement, in part by the stimulation of empathy created by the group process of problem solving. Another program, called Settle Conflicts Right Now (Osier & Fox, 2001), uses writing and drawing to stimulate empathy. By exchanging disclosures of upset feelings and problem solving, children become actively involved in the feelings of others and hence more empathic.

Effects

Although there are now many studies demonstrating that empathy can be taught, the challenging question of its effects on educationally relevant social and cognitive behaviors has been less thoroughly investigated. However, a number of studies and programs have directly assessed the effects of empathy training on other student behaviors.

The research described here addresses the training of empathy in an educational context and its social and cognitive effects. Lizarraga and colleagues (2003) addressed the effects of empathy training on self-regulation and self-control, attributes that are not usually included in analyses of the influence of empathy on education. Significant increments in self-regulation, self-control, assertiveness, and empathy were found in the empathy training group. Although the intervention was complex and the effects cannot be attributed solely to empathy, the theoretical relationship suggested between empathy and the self-regulation of emotions and behavior is of interest. A program that has been widely used in the United States and Canada since 1986, called Second Step, includes empathy as part of a violence prevention curriculum (Frey et al., 2005). Three components of empathy—recognizing feelings in self and others, considering others' perspectives, and responding emotionally to others—are the focus of the first unit of the Second Step Curriculum.

The Learning to Care Curriculum (Feshbach et al., 1984), designed for elementary-school-age children, consists of activities systematically related to one or more of the three components of the model of empathy described earlier (Feshbach, 1975, 1978). Activities include problem-solving games, storytelling, making tape and video recordings, and group discussion. Children who participated in the Learning to Care Curriculum became less aggressive, displayed more positive social behaviors, manifested a more positive self-concept, and also displayed a significant increase in academic achievement. Subsequent studies broadened the social objectives of empathy intervention (Feshbach & Konrad, 2001) and moved from the laboratory to the classroom (Feshbach & Rose, 1990). The approach was extended to problems of social prejudice in schoolchildren as well as aggressive behaviors (Feshbach & Feshbach, 1998).

The Citizen Curriculum, developed for middle-school students aged 9 to 14, is an activity-based teacher guide that is oriented toward building positive relationships. The primary focus of the program is the promotion of tolerance, empathy, and cooperation. Students role-play in a series of interactive workshops in which they discuss, debate, and problem-solve the challenges presented in the workshops (Hammond, 2006).

The promotion and training of empathy for the purpose of increasing tolerance and reducing prejudice would seem to be a logical endeavor. A potential stumbling block is the problem of implementing yet another program amid the already overburdened school day. A possible solution is to make empathy-enhancing procedures an integral part of the classroom's regular curriculum. The next study to be described offers a comprehensive and feasible method for integrating empathy into the school context.

The Curriculum Transformation Project

The Curriculum Transformation Project was an effort to apply empathy training to problems of social prejudice as well as aggression. An initial step entailed the development of principles for transforming the way in which standard curriculum is taught, with the goal of enhancing students' understanding and development of positive attitudes toward children from different ethnic and cultural backgrounds. At the same time, this curriculum transformation approach was intended to foster student's mastery of the curriculum content. A set of seven general transformational principles was developed to be applied to the instruction of regular classroom curriculum, in the areas of social studies, literature, composition, and art. The principles are presented in an appendix to this chapter.

A curriculum transformation program based on these principles was implemented for eight weeks in seventh- and eighth-grade social studies classes with primarily African American and Latino students (Feshbach & Konrad, 2001). After the eight-week period, the students in the curriculum transformation classes were rated higher in achievement and prosocial behavior and lower in aggression, while changes in empathy and social prejudice were negligible in all groups. With regard to social prejudice, the results varied widely. It is possible that classroom discussions of ethnic stereotypes and prejudices may temporarily elicit greater ethnic prejudice in some students.

Conclusions and Future Directions

The literature on empathy suggests that understanding of the process of empathy, in view of its potential for enhancing learning and social behavior, can make an important contribution to children's education. Empathy can be fostered through systematic training over a wide age range, from kindergarten children to adult teachers. However, a number of research gaps and challenges remain before the educational potential of empathy can be fully realized.

Many different procedures have been used to enhance empathy in teachers and in students, and it remains for systematic research and analysis to determine which interventions and which components of an intervention are most effective. Advances in cognitive neuroscience,such as research on mirror neurons, may provide a clearer understanding of the properties of empathy. The way empathy has been defined and measured in studies of teacher empathy differs from the way it has been assessed in most studies of empathy in students. Because of the numerous dimensions and varying definitions of empathy, its assessment may require multiple measures.

There is a need for additional research concerning the empathy training of teachers and its effects on student behavior and achievement. The teacher appears to be key to successful implementation over time of empathy training programs addressed to students. If teachers are directly involved in the empathy training of students, it is likely that the programs will be more successful.

It is clear that more research is needed to demonstrate the long-term effectiveness of empathy training programs in educational settings. At this point, it is fair to say that if teacher training programs impart knowledge of empathy and empathy training, such knowledge is likely to have positive effects on teachers and their students.

Appendix

Curriculum Transformation Project: General Transformational Principles

1. Where possible and appropriate, activities should be implemented that foster empathy, particularly toward individuals and groups that differ in race and ethnicity. Empathy can be enhanced through activities that increase students' sensitivity to and ability to identify feelings in others and in themselves, and their ability to take the perspective of others.
2. When the material in the curriculum involves instances of conflict, such as an argument or disagreement or fighting or war; of domination such as slavery, indentured servitude, and exploitation; or negative stereotyping such as labeling groups as inferior or unworthy, the students should engage in group discussions and other activities that lead to an understanding of the perspectives and feelings of the different individuals or groups involved.
3. Where possible and appropriate, similarities between individuals and groups that differ in cultural or other attributes should be emphasized. It is usually the case that while individuals and groups may differ in important respects, there are also important similarities.
4. Where possible and appropriate, when the material in the curriculum involves individual and group differences in appearance, customs, or values, it is important that the students, through group discussion and other activities, be helped to understand the significance of the difference. Some differences are superficial (e.g., food preferences); others may involve differences in perspective (how Marc Antony versus Brutus views the slaying of Caesar).
5. Where possible and appropriate, students should be encouraged through discussion and other activities to relate curriculum content to their own personal experiences.
6. Where possible and appropriate, students should be provided opportunities to appreciate features of their own background and ethnicity as well as to appreciate those of individuals with different backgrounds and ethnicities.
7. Where possible and appropriate, should the curriculum material or should children in the class cite negative actions of a particular ethnic group, the teacher may make use of the following principles:
a. All ethnic groups have engaged in negative behaviors.
b. There are individual differences within any ethnic group.
c. Historical circumstances may bring out the best and the worst in us.
d. Cultural standards and values change so that new generations may develop a different and often better sense of what is right and what is wrong.

e. Every generation has to work to bring about a better society; to bring about the best in themselves, in their ethnic groups, and in their nation; to reduce prejudice and violence; and to foster more constructive methods of resolving conflicts.

References

Aronson, E., & Patnoe, S. (1997). *The jigsaw classroom*. New York: Longman.

Aspy, D. N. (1971). Helping and intellectual functioning. In R. R. Carkhuff (Ed.), *The development of human resources, education, psychology, and social change*. New York: Holt, Rinehart & Winston.

Barak, A., Engle, C., Katzir, L., & Fisher, W. A. (1987). Increasing the level of empathic understanding by means of a game. *Simulation and Games, 18*, 458–470.

.Barnett, M. A., Howard, J. A., Melton, E. M., & Dino, G. A. (1982). Effects of inducing sadness about self or other on helping behavior in high and low empathic children. *Child Development, 53*, 920–923.

Barnett, M. A., Matthews, K. A., & Howard, J. A. (1979). Relationship between competitiveness and empathy in 6- and 7-year-olds. *Developmental Psychology 15*, 221–222.

Batson, C. D. (1991). *The altruism question: Toward a social psychological answer*. Hillsdale, NJ: Erlbaum.

Björkqvist, K., Österman, K., & Kaukiainen, A. (2000). Social intelligence – empathy = aggression? *Aggression and Violent Behavior, 5*, 191–200.

Black, H., & Phillips, S. (1982). An intervention program for the development of empathy in student teachers. *Journal of Psychology, 112*, 159–168.

Bonner, D., and Aspy, D. (1984). A study of the relationship between student empathy and GPA. *Humanistic Education and Development*, 149–153.

Brehm, S. S., Fletcher, B. I., & West, V. (1981). Effects of empathy instructions on first graders' liking of other people. *Child Study Journal, 11*, 1–15.

Budin, M. L. (2001). Tea and empathy. *School Library Journal 47*, 45–46.

Carkhuff, R., & Berenson, B. G. (1967). *Beyond counseling and psychotherapy*. New York: Holt, Rinehart & Winston.

Chang, A. F., Berger, S. E., & Chang, B. (1981). The relationship of student self-esteem and teacher empathy to classroom learning. *Psychology: A Quarterly Journal of Human Behavior, 18*, 21–25.

Chang, L. (2003). Variable effects of children's aggression, social withdrawal, and prosocial leadership as functions of teacher beliefs and behaviors. *Child Development, 70*, 535–538.

Cress, S., & Holm, D. T. (2000). Developing empathy through children's literature. *Education, 120*, 593–596.

Davis, O. L. Jr., Yeager, E. A., & Foster, S. J. (Eds.) (2001). *Historical empathy and perspective taking in the social studies*. Lanham, MD: Rowman & Littlefield.

Doyle, A. B., & Aboud, F. E. (1995). A longitudinal study of White children's racial prejudice as a social cognitive development. *Merrill-Palmer Quarterly, 1* (2), 209–228.

Eisenberg, N., & Miller, P. (1987). The relation of empathy to prosocial and related behaviors. *Psychological Bulletin*, 101, 91–119.

Feshbach, N. D. (1975). Empathy in children: Some theoretical and empirical considerations. *Counseling Psychologist, 5*, 25–30.

Feshbach, N. D. (1978). Studies on empathic behavior in children. In B. A. Maher (Ed.), *Progress in experimental personality research* (Vol. 8, pp. 1–47). New York: Academic Press.

Feshbach, N. D. (1998). Empathy: The formative years; Implications for clinical practice. In A. Bohart and L. S. Greenberg (Eds.), *Empathy and psychotherapy: New directions in theory, research and practice*. Washington, DC: American Psychological Association.

Feshbach, N. D., & Feshbach, S. (1982). Empathy training and the regulation of aggression: Potentialities and limitations. *Academic Psychology Bulletin, 4*, 399–413.

Feshbach, N. D., & Feshbach, S. (1987). Affective processes and academic achievement. *Child Development, 58*, 1335–1347.

Feshbach, N. D., & Feshbach, S. (1998). Aggression in the schools: Toward reducing ethnic conflict and enhancing ethnic understanding. In P. K. Trickett & C. J. Schellenbach (Eds.), *Violence against children in the family and the community* (pp. 269–286). Washington, DC: American Psychological Association.

Feshbach, N. D., Feshbach, S., Fauvre, M., & Ballard-Campbell, M. (1984). *Learning to care: A curriculum for affective and social development.* Glenview, IL: Scott, Foresman.

Feshbach, N. D., & Konrad, R. (2001). Modifying aggression and social prejudice: Findings and challenges. In H. Martinez (Ed.), *Prevention and control of aggression and the impact on its victims* 355–360. New York: Kluwer Academic.

Feshbach, N. D., & Rose, A. (1990). *Empathy and aggression revisited: The effects of classroom context.* Paper presented at the biennial meeting of the International Society for Research on Aggression, Banff, Alberta, Canada.

Feshbach, S., & Feshbach, N. D. (1969). The relationship between empathy and aggression in two age groups. *Developmental Psychology, 1*, 102–107.

Findlay, L., Girardi, A., & Coplan, R. J. (2006). Links between empathy, social behavior and social understanding in early childhood. *Early Childhood Research Quarterly, 21*, 347–359.

Frey, K. S; Nolen, S. B., VonSchoiack Edsrom, L. & Hirshstein, M. K. (2005). Effects of school-based social-emotional competence program: Linking children's goals, attributions and behaviors. *Journal of Applied Developmental Psychology, 26*, 171–200.

Hammond, A. (2006). *Tolerance and empathy in today's classroom: Building positive relationships within the citizenship curriculum for 9 to 14 year olds.* London: Paul Chapman Publishing.

Harbach, R. L., & Asbury, F. R. (1976). Some effects of empathic understanding on negative student behaviors. *Humanist Educator*, *15*, 19–24.

Higgins, E., Moracco, J., & Danford, D. (1981). Effects of human relations training on education students. *Journal of Educational Research*, *75*, 22–25.

Hietolahti-Ansten, M., & Kalliopuska, M. (1991). Self esteem and empathy among children actively involved in music. *Perceptual and Motor Skills*, *72*, 1364–1366.

Hoffman, M. L. (1982). Developmental prosocial motivation: Empathy and guilt. In N. Eisenberg (Ed.), *The Development of Prosocial Behavior*, (pp. 218–231). New York: Academic Press.

Hoffman, M. L. (1983). Affective and cognitive processes in moral internalization. In E. T. Higgins, D. N. Ruble, & W. W. Hartup (Eds.), *Social Cognition and Social Development: A Socio-Cultural Perspective* (pp. 236–274). Cambridge: Cambridge University Press.

Kalliopuska, M., & Ruokonen, I. (1993). A study with a follow-up of the effects of music education on holistic development of empathy. *Perceptual and Motor Skills*, *76*, 131–137.

Kelly, E., Reavis, C., & Latham, W. (1977). A study of two empathy training models in elementary education. *Journal of Instructional Psychology*, *4*, 40–46.

Kohn, A. (1991). Caring kids: The role of schools. Phi Delta Kappan, 72–7, 496–506.

Kremer, J. F., & Dietzen, L. L. (1991). Two approaches to teaching accurate empathy in undergraduates: Teacher intensive and self-directed. *Journal of College Student Development*, *32*, 69–75.

Lizarraga, L. S., Ugarte, M. D., Cardella-Elawar, M., Iriarte, M. D., & Baquedano, M. T. S. (2003). Enhancement of self-regulation, assertiveness, and empathy. *Learning and Instruction*, *13* (4), 423–439.

Lovett, B., & Sheffield, R. (2007). Affective empathy deficits in aggressive children and adolescents: A critical review. *Clinical Psychology Review*, *27*, 1–13.

Miller, P. A., & Eisenberg, N. (1988). The relation of empathy to aggressive and externalizing/antisocial behavior. *Psychological Bulletin*, *103* (3), 324–344.

Osier, J. L., & Fox, H. P. (2001). Settle Conflicts Right Now! A Step-by-Step Guide for K-6 Classrooms. Thousand Oaks: Corwin Press Inc.

Pecukonis, E. V. (1990). A cognitive/affective empathy training program as a function of ego development in aggressive adolescent females. *Adolescence*, 25, 59–76.

Perry, D. G., Bussey, K., & Freiberg, K. (1981). Impact of adults' appeals for sharing on the development of altruistic dispositions in children. *Journal of Experimental Child Psychology*, *32*, 127–138.

Redman, G. L. (1977). Study of the relationship of teacher empathy for minority persons and in service human relations training. *Journal of Educational Research*, *70*, 205–210.

Salovey, P., & Gruel, D., 2005. The science of emotional intelligence. *Current Directions in Psychological Science*, *14*, 281–285.

Sinclair, B. B., & Fraser, B. J. (2002). Changing classroom environments in urban middle schools. *Learning Environments Research, 5,* 301–328.

Stephan, W. G., & Finley, K. (1999). The role of empathy in improving intergroup relations. *Journal of Social Issues, 55,* 729–743.

Stout, C. (1999). The art of empathy: Teaching students to care. *Art Education, 52,* 21–24, 33–34.

Underwood, B., & Moore, B. (1982). Perspective-taking and altruism. *Psychological Bulletin, 91,* 143–173.

Warden, D., & Mackinnon, S. (2003). Prosocial children, bullies and victims: An investigation of their sociometric status, empathy and problem solving strategies. *British Journal of Developmental Psychology, 21,* 367–385.

Warner, R. E. (1984). Enhancing teacher affective sensitivity by a videotape program. *Journal of Educational Research, 77,* 366–368.

Yogev, A., & Ronen, R. (1982). Cross-age tutoring: Effects on tutors' attributes. *Journal of Educational Research, 75,* 261–268.

Zahn-Waxler, C., Radke-Yarrow, M., Wagner, E., & Chapman, M. (1992). Development of concern for others. *Developmental Psychology, 28,* 126–136.

Zeidner, M., Roberts, R. D., & Mathews, G. (2002). Can emotional intelligence be schooled? A critical review. *Educational Psychologist, 37* (4), 215–231.

III   Clinical Perspectives on Empathy

8   Rogerian Empathy in an Organismic Theory: A Way of Being

Jerold D. Bozarth

Empathy in psychotherapy emerged as a peripheral influence in classical psychoanalysis. Empathy in Freudian theory, most ostensibly, facilitated effective interpretations (Bohart & Greenberg, 1997, p. 9). However, Freud acknowledged empathy as indispensable for taking a position regarding another person's mental life (1921; cited in Decety & Jackson, 2004, p. 74). Empathy became a more central construct in psychotherapy when the processes of empathy were delineated by Reik and more recently as they have been considered relevant to the emerging field of social-cognitive neuroscience (Decety & Jackson, 2004, p. 74). Rogers's (1957) focus on empathy and unconditional positive regard as the core ingredients of therapy enhanced the role of empathy in psychotherapy and has turned out to be consistent with current conceptualizations in the field of social-cognitive neuroscience.

Client-Centered Theory

Client-centered therapy, developed by Carl R. Rogers, evolved to an organismic therapy in the 1950s (Rogers, 1959). It was initially developed as a theory of therapy in the late 1940s and early 1950s (Rogers 1942, 1951). At that time, it was often referred to as a *self* theory because of the centrality of the self-concept, self-experiences, and the ideal self to the theory. Empathy along with "warm acceptance" was considered the combined attitude critical to the therapeutic relationship. In developing his theory, Rogers concentrated on the therapist's method of "reflection" or "reflection of feeling" as empathic communication methods to facilitate the client's self-development (Rogers, 1942). Therapist responses were largely focused on in therapy sessions, research inquiry, and therapist/counselor training endeavors. Human Relations Training and Interpersonal Skills Training focused on operational definitions for levels of empathy (Carkhuff, 1969; Gordon, 1970) . The most current communication procedure in widespread use, known as Empathic Understanding Responses, offers a verbal response system that acknowledges therapists' attitudes (Brodley, 1997).

In 1951, Rogers shifted his emphasis from the mode of communication to the attitude of the therapist, noting: "The words—of either client or counselor—are seen as having minimal importance compared with the present emotional relationship which exists between the two" (Rogers 1951, p. 172).

The therapist's function was that of taking on "the internal frame of reference of the client, to perceive the world as the client sees it, to perceive the client himself as he is seen by himself, to lay aside all perceptions from the external frame of reference while doing so, and to communicate something of this empathic understanding to the client" (Rogers, 1951, p. 29). This idea evolved to a formal theory statement presented by Rogers in a 1955 University of Chicago Counseling Center discussion paper (Vol. 1, No. 5). The paper was published four years later and eventually proclaimed by Rogers to be "the most rigorously stated theory of the process of *change* in personality and behavior that has yet been produced" (Rogers, 1980. p. 59). The "conditions of the therapeutic process" were presented in succinct form:

1. That two persons are in contact.
2. That the first person, whom we shall term the client, is in a state of incongruence, being vulnerable, or anxious.
3. That the second person, whom we shall term the therapist, is congruent in the relationship.
4. That the therapist is experiencing unconditional positive regard toward the client.
5. That the therapist is experiencing an empathic understanding of the client's internal frame of reference.
6. That the client perceives, at least to a minimal degree, conditions 4 and 5, the unconditional positive regard of the therapist for him and the empathic understanding of the therapist (Rogers, 1959, p. 213)

These conditions were considered to be necessary and sufficient for therapeutic success and are identified as the therapeutic conditions in the theory of client-centered therapy. In combination, these conditions were also postulated as universal conditions for all therapies and helping relationships (Rogers, 1957). (Later, this theory was referred to as the "person-centered approach" in such contexts as education, administration, encounter groups, conflict resolution, management, community groups, and personal life [Rogers, 1977]).

The Organismic Influence of the Actualizing Tendency

Rogers's theory of client-centered therapy took a quantum leap, becoming a true organismic theory, with his formulation of "A theory of therapy, personality, and interpersonal relationships, as developed in the client-centered framework" (Rogers, 1959). Here, the client-centered approach was predicated on one motivational premise; namely, the *actualizing tendency* (Rogers, 1959, 1963). Later, Rogers included the *formative tendency*. This referred to a constructive direction "in the universe as a whole" (Rogers, 1980, p. 114). The formative tendency may have some pragmatic relevance in domains of the person-centered approach (e.g., community groups, education, encounter groups); however, the term is rarely included in theoretical discussions.

The actualizing tendency is "the inherent tendency of the organism to develop all its capacities in ways which serve to maintain or enhance the organism" (Rogers, 1959, p. 196).

In more pragmatic terminology, the process of client change can be described "as moving in the direction of actualization of their potentialities, moving away from rigidity and toward flexibility, moving toward more process living, moving toward autonomy, and the like" (Rogers, 1963, p. 8). To Rogers, the organism is viewed as "always motivated, always up to something, always seeking" (1963, p. 7). It is, however, only when the self-concept is congruent with organismic experiences that the constructive direction is facilitated; that is, organismic actualization and self-actualization must be synchronized. This is technically referred to as the *unitary actualizing tendency* (1963).

In 1951, the *self-actualizing tendency* was considered a positive directional force synonymous with the actualizing tendency. As Rogers noted, "The Self-Actualization of the organism appears to be in the direction of socialization, broadly defined" (Rogers, 1951, p. 488). The relationship of self-actualization and the actualizing tendency evolved to a more succinct meaning in Rogers's formal theory statement (1959). The therapeutic atmosphere would come to be defined by the client's experiencing of unconditional positive regard and empathic understanding as part of the therapist's congruence.

Empathy in Client-Centered Therapy

Empathy is embedded in the therapist's congruence. The actualizing tendency as a functional concept in therapy describes a person moving "away from rigidity and toward flexibility, moving toward more process living, moving toward autonomy, and the like" (Rogers, 1963, p. 8). Congruence is also described as the process of moving toward greater integration and development delineated by these characteristics. The hypothetical end point of this process is that of the "Fully Functioning Person" (Rogers, 1959, pp. 234–235). In short, empathy is part of the whole condition of congruence as a crucial condition for the therapist. Concomitantly, increased client congruence is the basic criterion of successful therapy for the client.

Rogerian empathy is different from all other concepts of empathy. As I have stated elsewhere, "The foremost reason for the difference of Rogers' concept of empathy from other concepts is that empathy for Rogers is intertwined with unconditional positive regard" (Bozarth, 1997, p. 8). For Rogers, empathy was also considered to be (1) a central therapeutic construct rather than a precondition to other forms of treatment, (2) an experiencing of the client rather than any particular therapist behavior, (3) a therapist attitude, and (4) an interpersonal process grounded in a nondirective attitude. Rogers defined empathy as follows: "The state of empathy, or being empathic, is to perceive the internal frame of reference of another with accuracy, and with the emotional components and meanings which pertain thereto, as if one were the other person, but without ever losing the 'as if' condition" (1959, p. 210). Rogers defined "empathy" in the theory but used the phrase "empathic understanding" in his formal statement. It is stated as condition five: "That the therapist is *experiencing* an *empathic* understanding of the client's *internal frame of reference*" (Rogers, 1959, p. 213; italics are in the original text and refer to words that are defined in the theory). The ultimate criterion for determining empathy (and unconditional positive regard) is the client's perception of this attitude (the sixth of the necessary and sufficient conditions).

Rogerian Empathy in Relation to Organismic Experiencing of the Client and Therapist

Rogers espoused client-centered therapy as an organismic theory and as a communication/interpersonal/self theory. These characterizations might complement each other, so that empathy is considered a complex form of psychological inference that combines observation, memory, knowledge, and reasoning (Ickes, 1997). However, emphasis on the therapist's communication can also hinder the expansion and exploration of the organismic theory. Hoffman's (1981) view of empathy, as primarily an involuntary vicarious response to affective cues, emphasizes a dimension more likely to be explained using neuroscientific frameworks. For example, Rogers (1959) omitted from his sixth condition of the therapeutic process the requirement that "the therapist *communicates* his empathic understanding and his unconditional positive regard to the client" (p. 213). He explicitly states that this was omitted "after much consideration" (p. 213). He explains: "It is not enough for the therapist to communicate, since the communication must be received . . . to be effective" (p. 213). The conflict that he struggled with is suggested by his explanation:

It is not essential that the therapist *intend* such communication, since often it is by some casual remark, or involuntary facial expression, that the communication is actually achieved. However, if one wishes to stress the communicative aspect which is certainly a vital part of the living experience, then condition 6 might be worded in this fashion: 6. That the communication to the client of the therapist's empathic understanding and unconditional positive regard is, at least to a minimal degree, achieved. (Rogers, 1959, p. 213)

The theory is consistent with the primary components—affective responding to another person, having cognitive capacity to take the perspective of another person, and having regulatory mechanisms of self—that are central to current investigations of empathy (Decety & Jackson, 2004).

In one of his rare revisions of the theory, Rogers (1975) elaborated upon the definition of empathy in an article titled "Empathic: An Unappreciated Way of Being." The main thrust of the revision was to frame empathy as a "process" rather than a "state." The change might be called a revision rather than a clarification, since the 1959 theoretical statement also referred to "being empathic" as well as to the "state of empathy" (Rogers, 1959, p. 110). Nevertheless, Rogers attempted to capture the quality of the empathic process with a more elaborate description. This elaboration actually adds little to the definition except by describing general activities of the therapist. Those activities include

1. The therapist entering the private perceptual world of the other;
2. The therapist being sensitive, moment by moment, to the changing felt meanings which flow in this other person;
3. The therapist temporarily living in his/her life, moving about in it delicately without making judgments;
4. The therapist communicating her sensings of the client's world;
5. The therapist frequently checking with the client regarding accuracy of these sensings, and being guided by the response received. (Rogers, 1975, p. 4)

Notably, there is a return to the emphasis on the therapist's communication including the periodic check of his or her accurate "sensings" of the client's frame of reference. Empathy is also referred to as an "unappreciated way of being," and as "dissolving alienation." It also helps the recipient to feel "valued, cared for, accepted as the person that he or she is." When this occurs, "true empathy is always free of any evaluative or diagnostic quality" (Rogers, 1975, pp. 6–7; Bozarth, 1999, p. 59). The nonevaluative and acceptant quality that Rogers ascribes to empathy is conceptually the same as his definition of unconditional positive regard, wherein the therapist experiences "a warm acceptance of each aspect of the client's experience as being a part of that client" (Rogers, 1957, p. 93; Bozarth, 1999, p. 59).

Rogers further commented about the therapeutic relationship a few years before his death in 1987. He contended that the client also participates in the empathic process of conscious-ness. As he put it, "I feel that in the best moments of therapy there is a mutual altered state of consciousness. That we really, both of us, somehow transcend a little bit what we are ordinarily, and there's communication going on that neither of us understands that is very reflective" (quoted in Heppner, Rogers, & Lee, 1984, p. 16).

The crucial pragmatic questions may be: When are clients experiencing empathic under-standing? And, how can this empathic understanding be measured? Some examples might help to explore these questions.

Clinical Scenarios

One way to consider when clients are experiencing empathy is to examine different client-therapist interactions that comprise empathic intentions. Determination of the extent of the therapist's experiencing of empathy in client-centered therapy lies exclusively in the client's perception (as stated in the sixth condition of the therapeutic process). Measurement has traditionally involved inventory tests and rating scales that take into account the perceptions of the therapist and those of objective raters as well as client perceptions. The Barrett-Lennard, Truax, and Carkhuff scales have been the most utilized among such mea-sures (Bohart & Greenberg, 1997, p. 16).

Several selected interactions from therapy sessions are offered in the following scenarios.

Pamela

The following vignette was presented more than twenty years ago (Bozarth, 1984).

The client was a graduate student, Pamela, who often sat in a catatonic state or continuously walked around on office furniture. This particular session, the therapist asked her what was "going on" when she entered appearing sullen and distant. She sat in silence for an hour and a half. During the session, the therapist said nothing but had a series of thoughts. The thoughts included: "I have complete faith in your resiliency to resolve your struggle." The therapist further thought to himself how Pamela might be feeling: "I feel so hurt and rejected. Did Harold reject you? It could have been several people or something else, but I think you feel Harold rejected you. But I know you don't want to talk about it." She got up and stood in a corner. The therapist thought: "What a bad girl am I."

She moved to behind a table and lay face down on the floor. Shortly, the therapist turned on a table lamp and turned on a tape with soft music while sitting in his chair next to Pamela. Twenty minutes later, Pamela said, "I have to go now," and went to the door. The therapist followed her asking: "Will you call me?" She responded with a pained look, "No."

Five minutes later, while the therapist was in a meditative state trying to assimilate the experience with Pamela, there was a knock on the door. It was Pamela saying, "I couldn't leave you like that." She started by saying that she was thinking of killing herself, but she changed her focus as she looked out the window of the fourth floor to see people walking below. "I wish I had a BB gun so I could shoot all of them," she said. "I wish it were a rifle," she continued, "so I could kill them all. Except the one there in a white blouse—I'd use an ax on her." The therapist questioned: "I don't get the ax for her?" The answer: "So it would be bloodier." Pamela continued her homicidal scenario describing the way she would go from floor to floor finding gory ways of destroying everyone. The therapist joined her several times saying, "Maybe a shotgun would be better . . . I'll remember not to wear a white shirt . . . " The session ended abruptly.

The next day, the therapist received a letter under his door from Pamela. She said: "(Today), I think 'silly me' I really would like to be calm and sane where Harold is concerned—what the hell makes him so important to me?" She went on to say that she was surprised that she could consider suicide, and described her discussion with a friend who said that she would be afraid that I would commit Pamela to a hospital. Pamela ended her letter by saying: "I am so aware of there being much more to life and by damn I want it. I'm so glad you didn't make those 'appropriate' responses that are so often so inappropriate. You really did understand me." (Bozarth, 1984, pp. 72–73)

Twenty years later, Pamela contacted the therapist. She was a successful entrepreneur and planning to return to graduate school to work on a doctorate degree. She indicated that she remembered our therapy sessions and still felt completely affirmed in the therapeutic relationship. According to her, the relationship and the empathic reception was one part of her successful life endeavors.

The incident contains a couple of examples of specific empathic interchanges in addition to Pamela's confirmation of being understood. The first consisted of the therapist's "sensing" that she was hurt by "Harold," a thought that was not even communicated to her. She confirmed this in her discussion when she returned to the session. A second nonconventional empathic experiencing was the interchange during the homicidal fantasy. She obviously relished my company in her world; no words of confirmation were needed.

In her letter to me the next day, she expressed her perception that I understood and accepted her. Twenty years later, she still offered the view that the empathic reception was a part of the relationship that helped her.

Tom

The context is slightly different in the next example because the therapy is described as "meditative therapy" and involved an experiment in which clinical students were to focus on clients in a way other than with words. The initial instructions directed the client to lie down and the therapist to sit beside the client. It was suggested that clients relax and, if they wished, tell the therapist what was going on with them at any particular time. The therapist was initially instructed to ask the clients periodically about what they were feeling, but also not to feel compelled to respond. I was the clinical supervisor and also served as therapist with several clients.

This scenario involves myself and one client. The client was a graduate student who was working on his doctoral degree in counseling psychology. He practiced meditation regularly on his own but wanted to meet with a therapist for specific help involving his marriage and vocational goals. He thought the meditation therapy might be a way for him to explore these goals. My experience with the experiment had evolved to simply sitting on the floor next to clients as they lay on a mat on the floor. Tom and I met for approximately a dozen sessions predetermined by the scheduled end of the university quarter. Tom explained at the outset that he wanted to meditate with someone present with him. He would "see what happens." He had major decisions to make regarding his marriage and career as well as anxiety about not completing his doctoral degree.

For twelve sessions, Tom came to the session, said "Hi," settled on the mat for an hour, then got up, saying, "Thanks." As the therapist, I focused on Tom and just allowed myself to experience whatever came to me. I generally did not think about anything. My focus was on Tom, in somewhat the way one focuses on a mantra. I directed my total attention toward Tom while allowing myself to experience whatever might occur.

A follow-up session with Tom revealed that his marriage had greatly improved; that he decided on a career direction; and that he had improved his school performance and decided to stay in school to finish his doctoral degree. Most of Tom's perceptions were confirmed by other sources as well.

The only substantial evidence of the therapist's empathic stance in this scenario was the therapist's intent to keep his attention on Tom. As the therapist, my feelings over the sessions moved from active and high-strung to calm and serene as the sessions unfolded. Unfortunately, measures of Tom's perception of empathy were not obtained. In the post-therapy interview, he did express that he was less "high strung" and had reached a calmness that he thought was essential to dealing with his specific concerns.

Jim

The following scenario is a small section from a therapy session of Carl Rogers with "Jim Brown" (Bozarth, 1996). Mr. Brown had been hospitalized in a mental hospital three times, the last time for 19 months. Rogers (1967) described the therapy sessions at length in the research project report. He met with Jim for 166 sessions of one hour or longer over a period of two and a half years. Rogers provided Mr. Brown with cigarettes, loaned him money, and sat in silence with him for most of the sessions. As Rogers summarized the process of therapy, "The progress he made appeared to grow primarily out of the qualities of the relationship. It appeared to have very little to do with fresh insights, or new and conscious self-perceptions. He became a new person in many ways, but he talked about it very little" (1967, p. 403).

I examined two of the therapy sessions in a previous review (Bozarth, 1996, pp. 240–250). I noted that the first session included 50 minutes of silence, two personal statements by Rogers, and eleven responses that were reflections with the intent of determining the meaning of Jim's statements. A couple of the responses were "empathic guesses," which Rogers indicated that he found himself periodically attempting in many of the sessions. These empathic guesses included the remarks "Do you look kind of angry this morning, or is that my imagination?" and "Sounds discouraged or tired." To the latter inquiry, Jim responded after a silence, "No, just lousy" (p. 244). When Rogers reflects an expression by Jim of feeling hurt by an acquaintance and feeling "no good," Jim defiantly responds by saying: "I don't care, though." Rogers responds: "You tell yourself you don't care at all, but somehow I guess some part of you weeps over it" (referring to Jim's tears). Rogers continues after 19 seconds with: "I guess some part of you feels, 'here I am hit with another blow, as if I haven't had enough blows like this during my life when I feel that people don't like me. Here's someone I've begun to feel attached to and now he doesn't like me. But just the same the tears run down my cheeks." (p. 245). A minute and a half go by in silence until Rogers responds to Jim's tears: "It really hurts, doesn't it?" Twenty-six seconds later, Rogers continues: "I guess if the feelings came out you'd just weep and weep and weep." After a little over a minute of silence, Rogers had to discontinue because of another appointment.

The second session, three days later, followed a similar pattern. There were 52 minutes of silence, 49 statements by Rogers of which 19 were reflections, and several empathic guesses. The guesses seemed to be directed more toward intensity of feelings than in the previous session. For example, Rogers guesses that Jim allows himself to "sink down into feelings that run very deep in you." However, Jim ignores these remarks with statements such as, "I'm gonna take off." Rogers responds with a reflection searching for more meaning and even uses a metaphor of "a wounded animal that wants to crawl away and die." Rogers continues with several personal statements, including one that he was feeling good about Jim not holding his hands over his face. Rogers considered one personal expression as the most meaningful statement of all of the sessions and viewed it as a "moment of movement" for Jim. The comment: "I think that I can understand pretty well what it's like to feel that you're just no damn good to anybody." . . . because there was a time I felt that way about myself. And I know it can be really rough.". As Rogers continued to respond to Jim, the "crucial turning point" came with the statement: "M-hm, m-hm. That's why you want to go, because you really don't care what happens. And, I guess I would just like to say—I care about you. And I care what happens." Jim burst into tears for the next fifteen minutes. Although there are several attempts more to engage Jim, he remains barely communicative the next few minutes of the session. Jim's final comment to Rogers was, "You don't have a cigarette, do you?" (Bozarth, 1996, pp. 245–246).

Mr. Brown got out of the hospital and was living a normal life several years after his discharge. Rogers believed that the crucial turning point was when Jim had given up and Rogers expressed his caring for Jim. Rogers summarized these interviews in the following way: "I felt a warm and spontaneous caring for him as a person, which found expression in several ways—but most deeply at the moment when he was despairing. . . . We were relating as two real and genuine persons" (Rogers, 1967, p. 411).

This example entails aspects of the three major functional components that interact to produce the experience of empathy in humans as it has been conceptualized through a multidisciplinary approach (Decety & Jackson, 2004). There is evidence of affective sharing of self by Rogers with Mr. Brown. It is also clear that Rogers maintained his own self-identity as he periodically entered Brown's perceptual world. Rogers sought to adopt Jim Brown's perspective in several ways. He listened intently and patiently to discussions about Brown's dissatisfaction with the hospital. Rogers periodically attempted "empathic guesses"; and he shared his own feelings regarding his caring about Jim. Notably, when Rogers verbalized his empathic guesses, Jim sometimes rejected the attempts, verbally correcting Rogers.

Discussion

Rogerian empathy is often associated with verbal empathic understanding responses (Brodley, 1997). In a verbal interchange the therapist can readily determine, by the client's response, whether empathic understanding has been communicated or whether an empathic attempt has been rejected or needs clarification. In the scenarios presented above, empathy is more difficult to identify because there is less verbal interaction. However, the criterion for determining the presence of empathy is the client's perception of unconditional positive regard and empathic understanding. Discrepant perceptions of empathy between the therapist and client are minimal since the fundamental activity of the therapist is to seek the client's perception of his or her life. The therapist is, in essence, always asking the client—in one way or another—whether or not the client's frame of reference is understood by the therapist.

As with other therapies, client-centered therapy can be assessed with measures developed by neuroscience. The more esoteric client scenarios in this chapter could give neuroscientists some ideas for examining empathy in similar therapeutic situations. For example, I wonder about examination of the brain activity of client and therapist using advanced technology during therapy sessions. How would the client's and the therapist's brain activity patterns compare at different junctures of the therapeutic process? For example, the extent of physiological correspondence of the therapist and Pamela during silences, or during her walking on the furniture, or during the therapist's companionship on her homicidal fantasy, could help to reveal the nature and extent of their psychological/physiological concordance. Such measures might have been useful to determine a more scientific basis for the therapist's sense of Tom moving from feeling "high strung" to greater calmness.

What if there had been extensive examination of the pulse rate, perspiration, and brain activity of Tom and the therapist during the span of the silent periods. Could there be a neurological determination that we perhaps know more than we think we know in the presence of another individual?

Three primary components of human empathy were identified by Decety and Jackson (2004) in their examination of its functional architecture. These components include the ability to share the emotional experience of another, the cognitive capacity to understand it, and the ability to simultaneously regulate one's own feelings; that is, to maintain the distinction between self and other's feelings. This discovery is notably consistent with Rogers's view of empathy. Although this chapter focuses on the organismic foundation of client-centered therapy and emphasizes the innate ability to experience the inner life of another, elsewhere Rogerian empathy has been embedded in the communication skill associated with verbal empathic understanding responses (Brodley, 1997).

Rogers stated more than once: "I recognize that when I am intensely focused on a client, just my presence seems to be healing and I think that this is probably true of any good therapist" (quoted in Baldwin, 1987, p. 45). Rogerian empathy could be better understood and further developed through the methods of social neuroscience. It is a long-standing and powerful concept that is compatible with the social-cognitive neuroscience model of inquiry.

References

Baldwin, M. (1987). Interview with Carl Rogers on the use of the self in therapy. In M. Baldwin & V. Satir (Eds.), *The use of self in therapy* (pp. 45–52). New York: Haworth Press.

Bohart, A., & Greenberg, L. (1997). *Empathy reconsidered: New directions in psychotherapy*. Washington, DC: American Psychological Association.

Boyer, P., & Barrett, H. C. (2004). Evolved intuitive ontology: Integrating neural, behavioral, and developmental aspects of domain specificity. In D. Buss (Ed.), *Handbook of evolutionary psychology*. Cambridge, MA: MIT Press.

Bozarth, J. D. (1984). Beyond reflection: Emergent modes of empathy. In R. Levant & J. Shlein (Eds.), *Client-centered therapy and the person-centered approach: New directions in theory, research, and practice* (pp. 59–75). New York: Praeger.

Bozarth, J. D. (1996). A silent young man: The case of Jim Brown. In B. A. Farber, D. C. Brink, & P. M. Raskin (Eds.), *The psychotherapy of Carl Rogers: Cases and commentary* (pp. 240–260). New York: Guilford Press.

Bozarth, J. D. (1997). Empathy from the framework of client-centered theory and the Rogerian hypothesis. In A. C. Bohart & L. S. Greenberg (Eds.), *Empathy reconsidered: New directions in psychotherapy* (pp. 81–102). Washington, DC: American Psychological Association.

Bozarth, J. D. (1999). *Person-centered therapy: A revolutionary paradigm* (2nd ed.). Ross-on-Wye, UK: PCCS Books.

Bozarth, J. D., Zimring, F., & Tausch, R. (2002). Client-centered therapy: Evolution of a revolution. In D. Cain and J. Seeman (Eds.), *Handbook of humanistic psychotherapy: Research and practice* (pp. 147–188). Washington, DC: American Psychological Association.

Brodley, B. T. (1997). The nondirective attitude in client-centered therapy. *Person-Centered Journal, 4* (1), 61–74.

Carkhuff, R. R. (1969). *Helping and human relations: A primer for lay and professional helpers: Vol. 1. Selection and training.* New York : Holt, Rinehart & Winston.

Decety, J., & Jackson, P. L. (2004). The functional architecture of human empathy. *Behavioral and Cognitive Neuroscience Reviews*, 3, 71–100.

Gordon, T. (1970). *T.E.T.: Teacher effectiveness training.* New York: New American Library.

Heppner, P. P., Rogers, M. E., & Lee, L. A. (1984). Carl Rogers: Reflections on his life. *Journal of Counseling and Development, 63*, 14–20.

Hoffman, M. L. (1981). Is altruism part of human nature? *Journal of Personality and Social Psychology, 40*, 121–137.

Ickes, W. (1997). *Empathic accuracy.* New York: Guilford Press.

Rogers, C. R. (1942). *Counseling and psychotherapy.* Boston: Houghton- Mifflin.

Rogers, C. R. (1951). *Client-centered therapy: Its current practice, implications, and theory.* Boston: Houghton Mifflin.

Rogers, C. R. (1955). A theory of therapy, personality, and interpersonal relationships as developed in the client-centered framework. *Counseling Center Discussion Papers, 1* (5), 1–69.

Rogers, C. R. (1957). The necessary and sufficient conditions of therapeutic personality change. *Journal of Consulting Psychology, 21* (2), 95–103.

Rogers, C. R. (1959). A theory of therapy, personality, and interpersonal relationships as developed in the client-centered framework. In S. Koch (Ed.), *Psychology: A study of science: Vol. 3. Formulation of the person and the social context* (pp. 184–256). New York: McGraw Hill.

Rogers, C. R. (1963). The actualizing tendency in relation to "motives" and to consciousness. In M. Jones (Ed.), *Nebraska Symposium on Motivation* (pp. 1–24). Lincoln: University of Nebraska Press.

Rogers, C. R. (1967). A silent young man. In C. R. Rogers, G. T. Gendlin, D. J. Keisler, & C. B. Truax (Eds.), *The therapeutic relationship and its impact: A study of psychotherapy with schizophrenics* (pp. 401–416). Madison: University of Wisconsin Press.

Rogers, C. R. (1975). Empathic: An unappreciated way of being. *Counseling Psychologist, 5,* 2–10.

Rogers, C. R. (1977). *Carl Rogers on personal power: Inner strength and its revolutionary impact.* New York: Delacorte Press.

Rogers, C. R. (1980). The foundations of a person-centered approach. In C. Rogers (Ed.), *A way of being* (pp. 113–136). Boston, MA: Houghton-Mifflin.

9 Empathy in Psychotherapy: Dialogue and Embodied Understanding

Mathias Dekeyser, Robert Elliott, and Mia Leijssen

In this chapter, we present an account of empathy in psychotherapy that is based on a more general, multidisciplinary understanding of everyday empathic interaction. We want to argue that, for two reasons, this approach can contribute to a better understanding of processes of empathy in the therapeutic context. Neurological studies and social psychology research have demonstrated the power and complexity of interpersonal influence on a physical, nonverbal level, a complexity that is sometimes ignored by therapists (Shaw, 2004). Examples of such influences are emotional contagion (e.g., Preston & de Waal, 2002) and automatic vigilance (Wentura, Rothermund, & Bak, 2000). Second, understanding problems in client-therapist interaction requires us to examine how clients both understand and misunderstand their therapists, including their therapists' intentions, emotions, and other internal states (e.g., Rhodes et al., 1994). These problems are grasped with more coherence when they are described using parallel concepts for the client and the therapist. For example, it is easier to understand and tackle severe communication problems in psychosis treatment when both the client's and the therapist's "sides" of the communication are considered (Peters, 2005).

The Empathy Cycle and Embodied Empathy

Empathy in the psychotherapy session is essentially a cooperative, dialogical process that is at the same time vividly grounded in the body, as illustrated in the following example (Bohart et al., 2002; Diamond, 2001; Wynn & Wynn, 2006).

Nick was an unemployed chef who came to therapy to deal with depression brought on by losing his job. In session three, he described what his work was like for him at its best and what he missed about it. As the therapist listened, he let himself be carried away into the client's experience: he felt a tickling, tingling sensation in his stomach; he remembered the feeling of his own similar successes (rising sense of excitement, accompanied by a sense of feet planted firmly on the ground); he "ran a movie in his head" of the client striding out of the kitchen, head held high, accompanied by a sense of pride and happiness. He noted how his fantasy matched Nick's upright posture and firm position in the chair, and how he had shifted into a firmer position himself. During his description, Nick felt that his therapist was interested and—even though the therapist had not said anything—he experienced support and an invitation to dig deeper into his description.

Empathy in psychotherapy is dialogical because it is based on the empathic faculties of both the client and the therapist, activated automatically through verbal and nonverbal exchanges, and enhanced by conscious efforts by each to understand the other. Although it involves perceptual, cognitive, and behavioral processes, it is fundamentally grounded in bodily and emotional experiences (Vanaerschot, 1990). Most of these elements have been incorporated in Barrett-Lennard's (1981) formulation of the Empathy Cycle (EC), still the most influential theory of professional empathic interaction (e.g., Elliott, Watson, et al., 2004). In the EC, client and therapist together search for an accurate expression of the client's experience, cycling through four steps: (1) client expression of experience; (2) therapist empathic resonation; (3) therapist expressing empathy; (4) client receiving empathy; followed by further client expression of experience. The EC model provides a clear, concise, and useful framework for understanding therapeutic empathy. *Empathic attunement* is presented as the therapist's internal representation of the clients' emotions, intentions, cognitions and physical states (step 2), which allows the therapist to respond (step 3) in a way that helps the client toward more accurate expression. Every new response by the client helps the therapist to better understand the client and allows the therapist to respond from a new, ever-deepening empathic stance.

Putting empathy in the bosom of the therapist, however, deflects attention away from its complement, the empathy of the client with the therapist, and also from the embodied nature of empathy. It is important to realize that most people resonate empathically with others. The effective monitoring of automatic interpersonal influences is a prerequisite for successful social interaction (Ickes, 2003; Decety & Jackson, 2004). Most relevant for our understanding of other people are the emerging feelings, thoughts, and responses of our own that are in line with their own behavior. Others' movements, eye contact, distance, breathing, and rhythm continuously prime similar motor responses in ourselves, as well as associated emotions, goals, and intentions (e.g., Chartrand & Bargh, 1999; Hood, Willen, & Driver, 1998; Iacoboni et al., 2005; Levenson & Ruef, 1992). Even our understanding of verbal expressions involves motor representations related to their meaning (e.g., Hauk, Johnsrude, & Pulvermüller, 2004). Yet each individual may react differently to this automatically induced convergence. When confronted with a seemingly calm but anxious person, one individual may unreflectively feel uneasy or annoyed. Another individual senses signs of fear in his own body and wonders whether this seemingly calm person is actually afraid. Only the second individual successfully performs *empathic resonance*.

We have begun to characterize dialogical, embodied empathy as a key concept in psychotherapy, at the same time arguing that it is not the exclusive province of community workers, nurses, or psychological therapists. Empathic resonance is naturally applied in every dialogue. For the rest of this chapter, we will elaborate the two sides of the empathic dialogue in the context of psychotherapy, beginning with the client's contribution.

Client Empathic Resonance

As clients explore their own intentions and motives, they long for the therapist's point of view, hoping to gain insight from that perspective even when it differs from their own. They not only value therapist empathy but also other therapist response qualities, and are therefore empathic partners themselves in their interaction with the therapist (Wynn & Wynn, 2006). Bänninger-Huber (1992), studying facial microsequences in clients and therapists, showed how clients carefully observe therapist responses in order to monitor their appraisal and the goal and direction of the interaction. When the client has problems resonating effectively with the therapist, then important therapist attitudes like empathy, acceptance, genuineness, and nonpossessive warmth (Lambert & Ogles, 2004) may not be noted. The therapist will have a difficult time engaging in an effective working relationship with the client, a condition critical to a positive therapy outcome (Horvath, 2001).

Client Empathy Problems

Interpersonal priming, self-awareness, mental flexibility, and emotion regulation constitute the macro components of internal empathy processes (Decety & Jackson, 2004). In addition, effective emotional expressiveness is required to communicate empathic listening. Even minor dysfunction in one or more of these component processes will fundamentally change interpersonal communication. In fact, empathy problems can arise in any client at any point of therapy, as client empathic resonance with the therapist is reduced by client expectations, a phenomenon known in psychodynamic theory as *transference*. For example, acute expectations of rejection or unresponsiveness from the therapist can lead to ruptures in the working alliance (Safran et al., 2005). Clients with such expectations may become withdrawn, demanding, or accusatory, triggering intrusive or attacking responses in the therapist. Most clients will now or then experience difficulties in maintaining a clear distinction between self and therapist, which often confuses the therapist (Diamond, 2001; Ross, 2000; Vanaerschot, 2004). More serious empathic failure has been reported for people who suffer neurological, psychotic, autistic, borderline, antisocial, and language disorders (Adams, 2001; Blair, 2005; Decety & Jackson, 2004; Ladisich & Feil, 1988), as well as for those who suffer from dementia (Dodds, Morton, & Prouty, 2004). In the more severe disorders the display of empathic resonance is very low (Krause et al., 1998), and the higher the symptom load, the lower the quality of the therapeutic relationship (McCabe & Priebe, 2003). It is much harder for the caregiver to develop a personal bond with such patients (e.g., Prouty, Van Werde, & Pörtner, 1998/2002; Vanaerschot, 2004).

Condition for Change

A non-body-oriented approach leads psychotherapists to limit their work to clients who are able to communicate verbally in a meaningful way. A central requirement for meaningful communication between two persons is that they can resonate effectively with each other. This mutual empathic resonance between two persons was termed "psychological contact" by Carl Rogers (1957), who considered it to be the most basic condition for therapeutic change. This position seems to support excluding from psychotherapy clients who don't communicate effectively. For example, cognitive therapy protocols for treating persons with psychosis or hallucinations require that the patient be able to discuss beliefs and attitudes with the therapist (Hermans & Raes, 2001). Even psychological interventions that aim to increase the empathic skills of clients generally focus on patients who are already performing at a moderately high level of communication (e.g., Alfred, Green, & Adams, 2004).

Yet, an empathic dialogue can occur whenever there is a minimal engagement from the client (Peters, 2005). Even infants try to engage in dyadic interaction, with properties of a dialogue gradually emerging (Stern, 1985; Gergely & Watson, 2002). Their engagement is apparent from the production of emotional responses, seeking of facial stimuli, gaze following, and attempts to imitate (e.g., Hood, Willen, & Driver, 1998). Peters (2005) argues that readiness for interaction is an inborn faculty that remains functional throughout life in all populations, including infants with an autistic spectrum disorder, psychotic adults, and older persons with dementia.

This view implies that an empathic process can be established with almost any client or patient, but only if the therapist can tune into the person's current, sometimes strange or frightening experiences and physical modes of expression (e.g., Killick & Allan, 2001). To accomplish this, Prouty, Van Werde, and Pörtner (1998/2002) advocate the use of *contact reflections* in these difficult-to-treat populations. These contact reflections are body-oriented, highly concrete, literal, and duplicative reflections that are at the same time explicit representations of the client's verbal and nonverbal behavior. For example, the therapist can say "Mary is sitting on the floor," or "Your arm is in the air." More concretely, the therapist can put his or her own arm in the same position. When applied consistently over time by one therapist or by all members of the staff on the ward (Van Werde, 2005), these responses expose the client to a "web of contact" that facilitates their own contact efforts.

Therapist Empathic Attunement

Although in most cases both client and therapist will naturally engage in empathic resonance, the therapist's engagement in empathy deserves a separate description. It is part of the therapist's task to resonate effectively with the client. *Empathic attunement* refers to the therapist's effortful engagement in empathic resonance (Bohart & Greenberg, 1997; Elliott, Watson, et al., 2004; Vanaerschot, 1990). Turning to the therapist side of the empathic process, we will now describe the phenomenology, functions, and effectiveness of empathic attunement.

Phenomenology of Therapist Empathy

When we teach empathic attunement, we begin with a phenomenological account of the therapist's experience of his or her own empathy. The starting point for this account is an understanding of empathy as essentially an imaginative, bodily experience rather than as a conceptual process. A wide range of language has been used to describe this experience, with five bodily metaphors capturing the major aspects: letting go; resonating; moving toward or into; discovering or discerning; and grasping or taking hold (Elliott, Watson, et al., 2004). Each of these metaphors provides only a partial approximation of the empathic attunement process; we offer them in order to provide a variety of potentially useful ways of understanding and developing this crucial attitude. A useful approach to deepening one's empathic stance is to successively apply these metaphors as an embodiment of the process of understanding clients.

The first aspect of the therapist's experience of empathy is captured by the image of hands *letting go*, a metaphor for setting aside preformed ideas, beliefs, or expectations, or previous understandings of the other (Vanaerschot, 1990). This image is reflected in language such as allowing, accommodating, suspending disbelief, bracketing (cf. Husserl's term *epoché*), or opening up. The therapist is aware of his or her views or preconceptions of the client and tries to let go of them in order to be more open to what the client is saying or revealing in the present moment. In addition, the therapist has to let go (temporarily) of current personal issues, for these will prevent a total opening up to the frame of reference of the client. To support this letting-go process, many therapists employ body-oriented awareness exercises in between sessions, thereby "clearing a space" for the experiences of the client (Nagels & Leijssen, 2004).

Second, the therapist seeks to actively *enter* the other's world, as evidenced by language having to do with moving toward or into the other. Thus, the therapist tries to join, become immersed in, dwell on, feel into (i.e., the source of the word "empathy"), or step under or inside (i.e., the origin of "understanding") the client's experience. Chartrand and Bargh (1999) and Sonnby-Borgström (2002) have demonstrated that persons who have the habit of taking other people's perspectives often mimic their postures, mannerisms, and gestures while listening to them. Some therapists will even perform stretching exercises before the session to increase their receptivity to client motor responses. Therapists may also actively "join" or "pace" the client by deliberately matching or trying out the client's verbal and nonverbal expressions, intensity, pace, or described internal sensations (Nagels & Leijssen, 2004). Beyond this, some therapists use touch to literally enter the client's space and get a direct physical sense of what the client is doing on a muscular level (Leijssen, 2006). In other words, in empathizing with the client, the therapist experiences an active reaching out in order to enter into the client's world. This may vary in degree from light interest and involvement with what the client is saying to intense states of "deep empathic immerse-ment" (Mahrer, 1989; Wertz, 1983).

Third, the therapist's experience of empathy includes the image of bodily *resonating* with the other (Barrett-Lennard, 1981), portraying the therapist as a tuning fork. This metaphor is reflected in language such as tuning in to, being "on the same wavelength," feeling with (i.e., compassion), feeling the same as (i.e., sympathy), singing in harmony with, or following or matching the client's experiencing. The therapist opens up to the sensations, actions, feelings, thoughts, and memories that well up in him- or herself while paying close attention to the client (Cooper, 2001). Therapists also feel an experiential understanding of underlying feelings different from those expressed explicitly by the client. For example, as her stomach contracts, the therapist finds herself sensing the fear that is covered up by the client's expressed anger. The moving toward and resonating experiences seem to complement one another: resonation is somewhat more receptive and entering-into is more active in nature. Given the central role of sensory perception in empathic resonance, it is no surprise that experienced therapists from many orientations maintain a body-oriented attention during sessions (Geller, Lehman, & Farber, 2002; Ross, 2000).

A fourth metaphor is the active, perceptual image of physically *sorting through* a large pile of something, discovering or discerning aspects of the other, finding, detecting, discriminating, pinpointing, or differentiating what is presented. This image captures the experience of complexity that often confronts the therapist. The therapist at times feels lost, confused, or overwhelmed by the sheer amount and variety of information revealed by the client. It often feels as if the important feelings or messages have been hidden or simply lost, like a needle in a haystack. In these situations, many therapists sustain bodily attention to discover a sense of direction (Gendlin, 1980; Nagels & Leijssen, 2004). The therapist's job is to see what is most crucial, pressing, or touching for the client.

A final image or component experience is that of actively *grasping* or taking hold of what is important in the client's world (Vanaerschot, 1990), as suggested by words such as apprehending, comprehending, getting (the point), assimilating, or perceiving. In other words, having entered into the client's world, the therapist then latches on to what is central, critical, alive, or poignant, sometimes with a sudden sense of insight into the other. The impression is one of taking some element of the client's experience inside oneself, thus making it part of oneself. On this basis, therapists will try to express what they think is important to the client, or they will respond in a way that makes sense from what they comprehend. When clients' responses are welcomed as continuous feedback for the process of attunement, empathic accuracy will increase (Marangoni et al., 1995).

Functions of Empathic Attunement in Therapy

Belief in the therapeutic value of empathic attunement was first put forward by humanistic psychologists, specifically Carl Rogers (1957), and it is still the cornerstone of the humanistic approaches to psychotherapy (Greenberg, Elliott, & Lietaer, 2003). Rogers proposed that a continuous effort by the therapist to empathically understand the client is necessary for therapeutic change to occur. This empathic attitude of the therapist is supposed to communicate a radical acceptance of client experiences, a condition that fosters self-acceptance and a more adequate, though sometimes painful, perception of oneself and one's life situation (Greenberg, Elliott, & Lietaer, 2003). In the humanistic and the psychodynamic tradition, the client is encouraged throughout most or all of the sessions to explore current or past experiences. The therapist can help to detect emerging experiences and what is deflected, while helping to regulate overwhelming or "fragile" experiences (Elliott, Watson, et al., 2004; Paivio & Laurent, 2001). This self-directed process is believed to lead to more accurate self-understanding and self-expression, more creative adaptation to current situations, a more effective way of interacting with others, a higher sense of self-agency, and ultimately to personality development (Bozarth, 2001; Greenberg, Elliott, & Lietaer, 2003).

In most schools of therapy it is now accepted that empathy is important for the formation of an effective working relationship (Castonguay & Beutler, 2005; Lambert & Ogles, 2004). Besides supporting the client's self-directed process, empathic attunement is an important way to manage therapist countertransference (Van Wagoner et al., 1991; Gelso & Hayes, 1998). In a classic psychoanalytic formulation, countertransference is the whole set of positive and negative feelings and responses related to the client (Heimann, 1950). Left unattended, these responses can hinder therapeutic progress. When they are explored properly by the therapist, however, they can offer a lead to individual and interpersonal processes that thus far remained implicit. Both empathic understanding (Decety & Jackson, 2004) and countertransference management (Gelso & Hayes, 1998) require the careful application of self-awareness, mental flexibility (discrimination between self and other), emotion regulation, and conceptualizing skills.

Therapist Empathy and Outcome

Bohart and colleagues (2002) conducted a meta-analysis of the available research relating empathy to psychotherapy outcome. Based on an exhaustive search of the literature, using previous reviews, research databases, and relevant journals, these authors located 47 studies, including 190 separate tests of the empathy-outcome association, and a total of 3,026 clients. Typically, these studies involved mixed, eclectic, or unspecified types of individual treatment, targeting affective and anxiety disorders. Client measures or observer measures of empathy were more generally used than therapist or accuracy measures of empathy. (Accuracy measures assess empathy by comparing therapist perceptions to client reports of their experience.) Pearson's correlation coefficient r was used as the measure of effect size, and various standard corrections for nonindependence and small sample bias were made, including pooling of effects within studies before averaging across studies.

The best estimate of the empathy-outcome association came from using data pooled within studies, weighted for sample size, and corrected for small sample bias: a mean r of .32. The size of this association was surprising, because it means that, in general, empathy accounted for about 10% of the variance in outcome, a medium effect size. This effect size is on the same order of magnitude found in previous analyses of the relationship between working alliance (between client and therapist) and outcome (e.g., .26 by Horvath & Symmonds, 1991; .22 by Martin, Garske, & Davis, 2000). Overall, empathy accounts for more outcome variance than does the specific intervention used. This value can be compared to Wampold's (2001) estimate that between 1% and 8% of outcome variance can be attributed to the mode of therapist interventions. Although this finding derives from a general sample of therapies, it provides a key line of converging evidence supporting the effectiveness of explicitly empathic therapies, such as person-centered and experiential approaches (Elliott, Greenberg, & Lietaer, 2004).

Perhaps empathy is even more important in an intervention-based therapy than in a relational one, in order to provide an effective "ground" for intervention. Bohart et al. (2002) found indications that empathy might be more important to treatment outcome in cognitive-behavioral therapies than in therapies that emphasize empathy. They also demonstrated that client measures of empathy predicted outcome the best, followed closely by observer-rated measures and therapist measures. In contrast, accuracy measures were unrelated to outcome. Ultimately, it seems that the client knows best whether the therapist is resonating effectively (Barrett-Lennard, 1981; Ickes, 2003; Rogers, 1957).

Finally, experienced therapists have been demonstrated to be both better at exploring their own experiences and better at interpreting clients' nonverbal behavior (Gesn & Ickes, 1999; Machado, Beutler, & Greenberg, 1999). Bohart et al. (2002) found larger associations between therapist empathy and treatment outcome for less experienced therapists, and a smaller association with outcome for more experienced therapists. It is possible that inexperienced therapists vary more in empathy, and that the smaller correlations for experienced therapists reflect a ceiling effect. Alternatively, experienced therapists may have developed additional helping skills (such as personal presence or effective problem-solving) that could compensate for moderate empathic misattunements.

Conclusion

We have attempted to outline a case for integrating the cognitive and affective approaches to empathy, grounded in the automatic convergence of physical states. We have attempted to go beyond a view of empathy as a conscious process of the therapist only, in order to sketch a view of empathy as fundamentally interpersonal. This dialogical, body-oriented perspective offers two main advantages: First, it highlights the continuity between therapy and other important human relationships and interactions, allowing us to draw on work in related disciplines. Second, it offers a richer, more complete understanding of empathy, highlighting client agency and providing important leads for therapy and therapy training. These leads include emerging directions for working with clients with severe communication difficulties, using body-based metaphors to learn deeper empathic responding, and drawing on one's body as a source of empathy. The dialogical, body-oriented perspective on therapeutic empathy is at the same time both more grounded in lived experience and better located in a wider human context of relationships and social interaction.

References

Adams, C. (2001). Clinical diagnostic and intervention studies of children with semantic-pragmatic language disorder. *International Journal of Language and Communication Disorders, 36*, 289–305.

Alfred, C., Green, J., & Adams, C. (2004). A new social communication intervention for children with autism: Pilot randomised controlled treatment study suggesting effectiveness. *Journal of Child Psychology and Psychiatry, 45*, 1420–1430.

Bänninger-Huber, E. (1992). Prototypical affective microsequences in psychotherapeutic interaction. *Psychotherapy Research, 2*, 291–306.

Barrett-Lennard, G. T. (1981). The empathy cycle: Refinement of a nuclear concept. *Journal of Counseling Psychology, 28*, 91–100.

Blair, R. J. (2005). Responding to the emotions of others: Dissociating forms of empathy through the study of typical and psychiatric populations. *Consciousness and Cognition, 14*, 698–718.

Bohart, A. C., Elliott, R., Greenberg, L. S., & Watson, J. C. (2002). Empathy. In J. C. Norcross (Ed.), *Psychotherapy relationships that work: Therapist contributions and responsiveness to patient needs* (pp. 89–108). New York: Oxford University Press.

Bohart, A. C., & Greenberg, L. S. (1997). *Empathy Reconsidered: New directions in psychotherapy*. Washington, DC: American Psychological Association.

Bozarth, J. D. (2001). An addendum to Beyond reflection: Emergent modes of empathy. In S. Haugh & T. Merry (Eds.), *Rogers' therapeutic conditions: Evolution, theory and practice* (Vol. 2, pp. 144–154). Ross-on-Wye, UK: PCCS Books.

Castonguay, L., & Beutler, L. (Eds.). (2005). *Principles of therapeutic change that work*. Oxford: Oxford University Press.

Chartrand, T. L., & Bargh, J. A. (1999). The chameleon effect: The perception-behavior link and social interaction. *Journal of Personality and Social Psychology, 76*, 893–910.

Cooper, M. (2001). Embodied empathy. In S. Haugh & T. Merry (Eds.), *Rogers' therapeutic conditions: Evolution, theory and practice* (Vol. 2, pp. 218–229). Ross-on-Wye, UK: PCCS Books.

Decety, J., & Jackson, P. L. (2004). The functional architecture of human empathy. *Behavioral and Cognitive Neuroscience Reviews, 3*, 71–100.

Diamond, N. (2001). Towards an interpersonal understanding of bodily experience. *Psychodynamic Counselling, 7*, 41–62.

Dodds, P., Morton, I., & Prouty, G. (2004). Using pre-therapy techniques in dementia care. *Journal of Dementia Care, 12* (2), 25–28.

Elliott, R., Greenberg, L. S., & Lietaer, G. (2004). Research on experiential psychotherapies. In M. J. Lambert (Ed.), *Bergin and Garfield's Handbook of psychotherapy and behavior change* (5th ed., pp. 493–540). New York: Wiley.

Elliott, R., Watson, J., Goldman, R., & Greenberg, L. S. (2004). *Learning emotion-focused therapy: The process-experiential approach to change.* Washington, DC: American Psychological Association.

Geller, J. D., Lehman, A. K., & Farber, B. A. (2002). Psychotherapists' representations of their patients. *Journal of Clinical Psychology, 58,* 733–745.

Gelso, C. J., & Hayes, J. A. (1998). *The psychotherapy relationship: Theory, research, and practice.* New York: Wiley.

Gendlin, E. T. (1968/1980). The experiential response. In E. Hammer (Ed.), *Interpretation in therapy: Its role, scope, depth, timing and art* (pp. 208–227). New York: Grune & Stratton.

Gergely, G., & Watson, J. (2002). The social bio-feedback model of parental affect-mirroring. In P. Fonagy, G. Gergely, E. L. Jurist, & M. Target (Eds.), *Affect regulation, mentalization and the development of the self* (pp. 145–202). New York: Other Press.

Gesn, P. R., & Ickes, W. (1999). The development of meaning contexts from empathic accuracy: Channel and sequence effects. *Journal of Personality and Social Psychology, 77,* 746–761.

Greenberg, L. S., Elliott, R., & Lietaer, G. (2003). Humanistic-experiential psychotherapy. In G. Stricker & T. Widiger (Eds.), *Handbook of psychology: Vol. 8. Clinical psychology* (pp. 301–326). Hoboken, NJ: Wiley.

Hauk, O., Johnsrude, I., & Pulvermüller, F. (2004). Somatotopic representation of action words in human motor and premotor cortex. *Neuron, 41,* 301–307.

Heimann, P. (1950). On counter-transference. *International Journal of Psycho-Analysis, 31,* 81–84.

Hermans, D., & Raes, F. (2001). De behandeling van wanen en hallucinaties: Gedragsanalytische en cognitieve benaderingen. *Gedragstherapie, 34,* 181–204.

Hood, B. M., Willen, J. D., & Driver, J. (1998). Adult's eyes trigger shifts of visual attention in human infants. *Psychological Science, 9,* 131–134.

Horvath, A. O. (2001). The alliance. *Psychotherapy: Theory, Research, Practice, Training, 38,* 365–372.

Horvath, A. O., & Symmonds, B. D. (1991). Relation between working alliance and outcome in psychotherapy: A meta-analysis. *Journal of Counseling Psychology, 36,* 223–233.

Iacoboni, M., Molnar-Szakacs, I., Gallese, V., Buccino, G., Mazziotta, J. C., & Rizzolatti, G. (2005). Grasping the intentions of others with one's own mirror neuron system. *Public Library of Science Biology, 3,* 529–535.

Ickes, W. (2003). *Everyday mind reading: Understanding what other people think and feel.* Amherst, NY: Prometheus Books.

Killick, J., & Allan, K. (2001). *Communication and the care of people with dementia.* Buckingham, UK: Open University Press.

Krause, R., Steimer-Krause, E., Merten, J., & Ulrich, B. (1998). Dyadic interaction regulation, emotion and psychopathology. In W. F. Flack, Jr., & J. D. Laird (Eds.), *Emotions in psychopathology: Theory and research* (pp. 70–80). New York: Oxford University Press.

Ladisich, W., & Feil, W. B. (1988). Empathy in psychiatric patients. *British Journal of Medical Psychology, 61*, 155–162.

Lambert, M. J., & Ogles, B. M. (2004). The efficacy and effectiveness of psychotherapy. In M. J. Lambert (Ed.), *Bergin and Garfield's handbook of psychotherapy and behavior change* (5th ed., pp. 139–193). New York: Wiley.

Leijssen, M. (2006). Validation of the body in psychotherapy. *Journal of Humanistic Psychology, 64*, 126–146.

Levenson, R. W., & Ruef, A. M. (1992). Empathy: A physiological substrate. *Journal of Personality and Social Psychology, 63*, 234–246.

Machado, P. P., Beutler, L. E., & Greenberg, L. S. (1999). Emotion recognition in psychotherapy: Impact of therapist level of experience and emotional awareness. *Journal of Clinical Psychology, 55*, 39–57.

Mahrer, A. (1989). *How to do experiential psychotherapy.* Ottawa: University of Ottawa Press.

Marangoni, C., Garcia, S., Ickes, W., & Teng, G. (1995). Empathic accuracy in a clinically relevant setting. *Journal of Personality and Social Psychology, 68*, 854–869.

Martin, D. J., Garske, J. P., & Davis, M. K. (2000). Relation of the therapeutic alliance with outcome and other variables: A meta-analytic review. *Journal of Consulting and Clinical Psychology, 68*, 438–450.

McCabe, R., & Priebe, S. (2003). Are therapeutic relationships in psychiatry explained by patients' symptoms? Factors influencing patient ratings. *European Psychiatry, 18*, 220–225.

Nagels, A., & Leijssen, M. (2004). De benadering van het lichaam in experiëntiële psychotherapie. In N. Stinckens & M. Leijssen (Eds.), *Wijsheid in cliëntgericht-experiëntiële gesprekstherapie* (pp. 63–82). Leuven, Belgium: Leuven University Press.

Paivio, S. C., & Laurent, C. (2001). Empathy and emotion regulation: Reprocessing memories of childhood abuse. *Journal of Clinical Psychology, 57*, 213–226.

Peters, H. (2005). Pre-therapy from a developmental perspective. *Journal of Humanistic Psychology, 45*, 62–81.

Preston, S. D., & de Waal, F. B. M. (2002). Empathy: Its ultimate and proximate bases. *Behavioral and Brain Sciences, 25*, 1–72.

Prouty, G., Van Werde, D., & Pörtner, M. (1998/2002). *Pre-therapy: Reaching contact-impaired clients.* Ross-on-Wye, UK: PCCS Books.

Rhodes, R. H., Hill, C. E., Thompson, B. J., & Elliott, R. (1994). Client retrospective recall of resolved and unresolved misunderstanding events. *Journal of Counseling Psychology, 41*, 473–483.

Rogers, C. R. (1957). The necessary and sufficient conditions of therapeutic personality change. *Journal of Consulting Psychology, 21*, 95–103.

Ross, M. (2000). Body talk: Somatic countertransference. *Psychodynamic Counselling, 6*, 451–467.

Safran, J. D., Muran, J. C., Samstag, L., & Winston, A. (2005). Evaluating an alliance focused treatment for potential treatment failures. *Psychotherapy, 42*, 512–531.

Shaw, R. (2004). The embodied psychotherapist: An exploration of the therapist's somatic phenomena within the therapeutic encounter. *Psychotherapy Research, 14*, 271–288.

Sonnby-Borgström, M. (2002). Automatic mimicry reactions as related to differences in emotional empathy. *Scandinavian Journal of Psychology, 43*, 433–443.

Stern, D. N. (1985). *The interpersonal world of the infant.* New York: Basic Books.

Vanaerschot, G. (1990). The process of empathy: Holding and letting go. In G. Lietaer, J. Rombauts, & R. Van Balen (Eds.), *Client-centered and experiential psychotherapy in the nineties* (pp. 269–293). Leuven, Belgium: Leuven University Press.

Vanaerschot, G. (2004). It takes two to tango: On empathy with fragile processes. *Psychotherapy: Theory, Research, Practice, Training, 41*, 112–124.

Van Wagoner, S., Gelso, C. J., Hayes, J. A., & Diemer, R. (1991). Countertransference and the reputedly excellent therapist. *Psychotherapy, 28*, 411–421.

Van Werde, D. (2005). Facing psychotic functioning: Person-centred contact work in residential psychiatric care. In S. Joseph & R. Worseley (Eds.), *Person-centered psychopathology: A positive psychology of mental health* (pp. 158–168). Ross-on-Wye, UK: PCCS Books.

Wampold, R. E. (2001). *The great psychotherapy debate: Models, methods, and findings.* London: Erlbaum.

Wentura, D., Rothermund, K., & Bak, P. (2000). Automatic vigilance: The attention-grabbing power of approach- and avoidance-related social information. *Journal of Personality and Social Psychology, 78*, 1024–1037.

Wertz, F. J. (1983). From everyday to psychological description: Analyzing the moments of a qualitative data analysis. *Journal of Phenomenological Psychology, 14*, 197–241.

Wynn, R., & Wynn, M. (2006). Empathy as an interactionally achieved phenomenon in psychotherapy. *Journal of Pragmatics, 38*, 1385–1397.

10 Empathic Resonance: A Neuroscience Perspective

Jeanne C. Watson and Leslie S. Greenberg

For decades, psychoanalytic, humanistic, and cognitive-behavior theorists have all emphasized the role of therapeutic empathy in facilitating change in psychotherapy. Most theorists have focused primarily on the function and expression of empathy. Some schools see it as a facilitative condition; others consider it a more essential ingredient of change. Less emphasis has been placed on what novice and experienced therapists can do to enhance their empathic skills. But recent developments in cognitive neuroscience have provided more insights into the nature of empathy and its various component processes. These insights suggest ways of refining our understanding of the construct so that therapists' empathic capacities to facilitate clients' changes in psychotherapy can be developed and enhanced.

Humanistic therapists see empathy as an active change agent in psychotherapy (Barrett-Lennard, 1993; Bohart & Greenberg, 1997; Bozarth, 1997; Elliott et al., 2003; Greenberg & Watson, 2006; Rogers, 1965; Warner, 1997). For Rogers (1965) empathy was both an emotional and a cognitive process, defined as the ability to perceive accurately the internal frames of reference of others in terms of their meanings and emotional components—as if one were the other, but without ever losing the "as if" condition. Rogers conceived of empathy as an attempt to actively experience clients' feelings, and to try to get under their skin. It is an attempt to absorb the meanings and attitudes of the other (Rogers, 1951). Rogers was careful to distinguish identification from empathy, seeing the former as indicative of a loss of boundaries. He suggested that the provision of empathy in psychotherapy allowed clients the opportunity to explore and reflect on themselves, thereby facilitating self-directed change.

Barrett-Lennard (1993) described therapeutic empathy as an active, cyclical process characterized by three phases: empathic resonance, empathic communication, and the resulting received or perceived empathy. First, therapists resonate to their clients' experiences, using their own bodies and inner experience to understand how their clients feel about their experience and what it means to them; second, therapists communicate their understanding to their clients; and third, clients have to receive their therapists' empathy so that they are aware of being understood.

Empathy and Neuroscience

Research has focused on whether and how empathy affects client change in psychotherapy. Less attention has been paid to the process of empathic resonance. Recent findings from cognitive neuroscience suggest that the ways in which empathy has been conceptualized by humanistic and psychoanalytic writers bears some resemblance to the cognitive and affective processes that are activated when people experience empathy. Neuroscientists define empathy as a "complex form of psychological inference that enables us to understand the personal experiences of another person through cognitive, evaluative and affective processes" (Danziger, Prkachin, & Willer, 2006). Storytellers, filmmakers, musicians, and advertisers have known and capitalized on our innate capacity to resonate to the feelings of others for a long time; however, for the first time we are able to map the physiological correlates of the processes of empathy, describe its neuronal architecture, and specify empathy circuits in the brain (Rankin et al., 2006; Ferrari et al., 2003). The technology that has allowed us to image the brain and identify different areas of activation during different activities has created an important window that is beginning to illuminate the links between psychological theories, experiential knowledge, empathic understanding, and physical processes. One of the major findings from brain mapping is the discovery of mirror neurons, which was heralded as one of the most exciting recent events in neuroscience.

Research on mirror neurons shows that similar brain regions are activated in an observer as those activated in a person who is experiencing a particular sensation—such as pain, sound, or touch—or performing certain actions (Rankin et al., 2006). Gazzola, Aziz-Zadeh, and Keysers (2006) found that auditory mirror neurons were activated when monkeys performed an auditory task, when they listened to an auditory task being performed, and when they saw an auditory task being performed. Thus the process of observing or imagining produces representations of that state in an observer or in one imagining the task being performed. This phenomenon is relevant to emotional processing as well. Regions in the brain associated with feeling a specific emotion are activated by seeing that emotion in another or witnessing the other in a situation that might elicit the emotion. It is important to note that these reproductions are not one-to-one simulations. Certain areas of the brain that would alert us to our own personal experience are not activated in observers, thus preserving the "as if" condition that Rogers (1965) and other psychotherapists have emphasized in their writings on empathy.

A review of the neuroscience literature on empathy reveals a number of important findings that have particular relevance for psychotherapy practitioners: First, mirror neurons provide the ability to understand the actions of others; second, people have an innate ability to imitate others; third, the context in which actions occur is vital to understanding and interpreting others' actions; fourth, responses to others' pain can be self-oriented or other-oriented; and fifth, there is neurological evidence that individuals differ from one another in their capacity to empathize.

Some investigators have suggested that the discovery of mirror neurons has begun to provide a physiological underpinning to theories of mind. Research to date indicates that empathy is hardwired, that it is an innate capacity whose precursors are evident from birth (Decety & Jackson, 2004). Infants and toddlers have been shown to be able to extrapolate the intentions of others. By observing the actions of others, infants and toddlers can complete tasks that have been started and give correct performances of tasks that they have been shown with errors (Decety & Jackson, 2004). These findings suggest that people are hard-wired to develop theories of mind with respect to themselves and other people and that this capacity is an important basis of social interaction and communication.

Mirror neurons do not fire indiscriminately; instead, firing is limited to goal-directed actions (Ferrari et al., 2003). The firing of mirror neurons in response to the goal-directed actions of others informs the observer of the intentions of the other, thereby illuminating the emotional and motivational significance of the observed acts. Wilson & Knoblich (2005) noted that action understanding is based on first being able to recognize and categorize specific actions; second, grasping the teleological and goal-directed objectives of other people's actions; and third, representing the mental state of others. These capacities enable us to project actions forward and anticipate what will happen in the future. A study by Gazzola, Aziz-Zadeh, and Keysers (2006) suggests a link between individuals' motor mirror systems and empathy. They found that individuals who score higher on a self-report measure of empathy show a stronger activation of their auditory mirror neurons than those who score lower.

The neural underpinnings of empathy are likely to be widely distributed and encompass the emotional parts of the brain, including the anterior cingulate cortex, insula, thalamus, and somatosensory cortices, as well as the right inferior parietal lobe (Meltzoff & Decety, 2003; Ferrari et al., 2003). The right inferior parietal cortex is thought to play a key role in humans' capacity to identify with others by apprehending their subjective states. Moreover, different areas of the brain are activated depending on whether a first- or third-person perspective is taken.

Studies that examine how people respond to watching others in pain reveal brain activation in areas associated with the emotional content of pain but not with the pain itself (Danziger, Prkachin, & Willer, 2006; Morrison et al., 2004; Jackson, Meltzoff, & Decety, 2005; Singer et al., 2004). Thus when we empathize we are simulating some aspects of another's experience within ourselves but not all aspects, as we are not experiencing the pain (Preston & de Waal, 2002; Singer et al., 2004). Observing and watching others in a particular emotional state automatically activates a representation of that state in the observer, with its associated autonomic and somatic responses (Preston & de Waal, 2002). This process can be activated through actual observation, listening to stories, visualizing, or imagining various scenarios (Danziger, 2006; Jackson & Decety, 2004), though there may be differences in the evoked potentials for each modality. For example, Jackson and Decety (2004) reported that imagining has a lower evoked potential than observing, and that film-generated emotion and recall-generated emotion have symmetrical increases in activation in the medial prefrontal cortex and the thalamus. Observing films leads to the activation of the hypothalamus, amygdala, anterior temporal cortex, and occipitotemporoparietal junction. Similarly, regions associated with feeling an emotion are activated by seeing the facial expression of the same emotion. This may be a similar process to that which enables us to produce feelings by adopting the facial expressions and postures associated with those feelings. Although empathy relies on body movements, they are not necessary; empathy can occur independently of motor network activation (de Vignemont & Singer, 2006).

Ways of Enhancing Therapists' Empathic Capacity

Neuroscience research on the physiological correlates of empathy provides support for therapists' subjective experience of trying to be empathic in a session and suggests ways in which therapists can heighten and enhance their empathic skills. Therapists can engage in a number of cognitive-affective processes to maximize their empathic capacity with their clients. First, therapists can use visualization techniques and actively imagine the experiences and events in their clients' lives; second, therapists can pay close attention to their bodies to discern the feelings or sensations that are being activated; third, therapists can listen carefully to the details and context of clients' life experiences; fourth, therapists can strive to decenter from their own experience to take on the perspective of the other; fifth, therapists can cultivate self-awareness and self-reflection; and sixth, therapists can learn to correctly identify other people's emotions from their narratives and nonverbal behavior. Research by Greenberg and Rushanski-Rosenberg (2002) into the subjective experience of expert therapists as they try to empathically resonate to their clients' experience suggests that they are engaging in these activities to enhance their empathic capacity. However, by mastering and attending to these specific processes more consciously, therapists may be better able to resonate and express their empathic understanding within a session. Each of these processes and the neurological research that supports them are reviewed here.

Visualization

The important role that visualization plays in the empathic process is illuminated by research on mirror neurons in observers that mimic the intentions, sensations, and emotions of those around them (Ferrari et al., 2003; Rizzolatti, 2005; Gallese, 2005). Decety and Jackson (2004) note that deliberate acts of imagination produce stronger responses in the neuronal empathy circuit than observation alone. Thus one way therapists could heighten their understanding of another person's state is by actively visualizing the details of the story they are being told. Therapists can try to develop mental images of different situations. It is likely that amplifying their responses will provide therapists with a better sense of what is happening for clients than passively listening to their tales and life experience.

Mimicry

As recorders of actions, mirror neurons are also seen as the precursors of mimicry. They not only allow us to receive and decode the actions and intentions of others but can facilitate communication with others to the extent that automatic mimicking of the actions of others indicates that we see them and can follow their stories (Wilson & Knoblich, 2005). When people see actions performed, the firing of mirror neurons stimulates similar physiological processes in the observer, providing them with a sense of the experience similar to that of the doer. Therapists who attend to their own covert experience of imitating their clients' actions can gain a better sense of what their clients might be experiencing. Therapists can then feed this information back to clients in order to communicate empathy with their experience and thus help them to verbalize it.

Another way therapists can use the automatic capacity to mimic others to help feel themselves into their clients' experience is to imitate their clients more overtly in the session and ask them what they are communicating with their actions. More overt imitation can heighten clients' awareness of their emotions and help them and their therapists to find the words to express and label their subjective states more clearly (Elliott et al., 2003; Kennedy-Moore & Watson, 1999). Alternatively, by attending to the covert process of imitation that is stimulated by visualizing another's actions or imagining oneself in the place of another, therapists can extrapolate from this activity and tentatively offer empathic conjectures to their clients about their emotional experience.

To the extent that analogous states are reproduced in observers, the body is an important source of information about how different experiences impact others. Therapists can use their knowledge of their own bodies to imagine what it must be like to be in different situations and experience certain things as they listen to their clients' narratives. This will help them feel themselves into their clients' worlds. Wilson & Knoblich (2005) suggested that, as a result of the activation of motor mirror neurons, we are able to use the implicit knowledge of our own bodies to track another's action. He proposed a perceptual emulator model whereby activation of motor neurons through observation, visualization, or listening results not only in the activation of mirror neurons but also in the ability to predict others' actions.

Context

Research has indicated that neural circuits are not automatically activated but respond selectively depending on the context (Wilson & Knoblich, 2005). Iacoboni and his colleagues have shown that mirror neurons fire differentially depending on the situation in which actions are embedded (Iacoboni et al., 2005). The researchers showed participants three different videos of a hand picking up a teacup. In the first video, the teacup was set on a table next to a teapot and a plate of cookies, indicating that a tea party was in progress; in the second video, the teacup was sitting on a table that was messy and scattered with crumbs; and in the third video, the teacup was sitting on a table without any other objects around it. The mirror neurons of participants shown these pictures responded more strongly to the teacup in the context of a tea party than they did to the scene without any other cues with respect to context. This result suggests that people interpret and understand others' actions in terms of the context in which they occur.

If therapists are to be maximally empathic, it is important for them to have a sense of their clients' current and past contexts and life histories in order to build an adequate understanding of what is emotionally significant for them and to gain an understanding of what motivates their actions. Humanistic therapists have tended to emphasize moment-to-moment responding in the session and have placed less emphasis on obtaining full accounts of clients' life histories. At times clients' attempts to tell their stories may be viewed as counterproductive in experiential psychotherapy; it is sometimes considered a distraction from their emotional processing. This view contrasts with that of analytic theorists, who emphasize the need for historical detail.

Given the importance of context for our brains to respond empathically to different situations, it is likely that to be maximally empathic therapists require a very good sense of the specific situations that have contributed to their clients' feeling and acting in the ways that they do. Therapists can attend to the quality of clients' stories. Experiential therapists have been aware that the manner in which clients tell their stories is an important marker of their emotional processing in a session (Elliott et al., 2003; Watson & Bohart, 2001). Experiential therapists listen to whether their clients are giving rehearsed descriptions of scenes or are rambling. At these times experiential therapists try to help clients get more in touch with their emotional processing. One way they do this is by asking clients to give more detailed, specific, and vivid accounts of situations. These descriptions provide an inside view of the clients' worlds, enabling therapists to develop a better sense of what their clients are feeling. They can then offer this conjecture to their clients to help them get more in touch with their emotions.

Obtaining an inside view and a clear sense of clients' narratives may be as important for therapists' processing in the session as it is for clients. By listening to detailed, vivid, and clear stories, therapists are more likely to be able to be empathic to their clients' experience and come to a better understanding of their worldviews. To enhance empathic resonance, therapists can ask clients for the details of situations to get a better sense of the contexts of clients' lives, or they might suggest systematic evocative unfolding—helping clients to "play a movie of a scene"—so that situations come alive for both participants in the session (Rice & Saperia, 1984; Watson & Rennie, 1994; Watson & Greenberg, 1996). More recently, experiential therapy researchers have recognized the importance of obtaining life histories and identifying the emotionally live and salient events and situations in clients' lives. This facilitates case formulation by providing an understanding of the emotional significance of specific events and the reasons clients feel and act the way they do (Watson, Goldman, & Greenberg, 2007).

Decentering

Researchers who investigate individuals' responses to others in pain have observed that responses can be self-oriented or other-oriented, varying along a continuum from personal agitation at the state of another to full understanding of the other's experiences. Jackson, Meltzoff, and Decety (2005) suggested that human beings' default mode is egocentric; however, the expression of empathy toward others requires the capacity to decenter. Merging can result in emotional contagion, wherein people experience and express distress at another's distress but do not fully comprehend the experience of the other. In order to fully comprehend another's experience it is important to remain differentiated, although it is clear that even when agitated the brain is able to distinguish personal pain from the pain of others. Studies of those individuals who showed responses to other people's pain indicated that different areas of the brain respond depending on whether the individual is the subject or the observer of painful experiences (Jackson, Meltzoff, & Decety 2005).

Gazzola and colleagues (2006) found that those individuals who had higher scores on a self-report measure of perspective taking showed greater activation of their auditory mirror neuron systems when they heard, saw, or imagined someone performing an auditory act. Interestingly, other subscales of the empathy measure including, empathic concern, the capacity to fantasize, and personal distress, did not correlate with the activation of mirror neurons. Instead, empathic concern was correlated with insula activation, which suggests that it is important to distinguish the cognitive and emotional aspects of empathy. Cognitive empathy and getting a sense of how another person is feeling or what they are experiencing may be linked to the capacity to take the perspective of another; it is likely to be different from concern or feeling distress at another's pain. Moreover, it appears that a personal experience of pain is not necessarily required for perceiving another's pain and feeling empathy (Danziger, 2006). The activation of specific neural networks seems to indicate that individuals are able to recognize events that might be painful to others and register others' responses to painful events (de Vignemont & Singer, 2006), leading some researchers to suggest that different aspects of empathy may depend on different neural substrates (Gazzola et al., 2006; Jackson et al., 2006).

As psychotherapists have noted, the experience and expression of empathy does not require merging with others (Jackson et al., 2006). Rather, a capacity to decenter seems to be essential for people to be able to fully empathize with the experiences of another. When Rogers first started writing about empathy in psychotherapy, he emphasized the need for therapists to be nonjudgmental and accepting of their clients' experiences. For therapists to be truly nonjudgmental, Rogers suggested that they must put aside their own perspectives, worldviews, values, and preferences as they try to fully enter their clients' worlds and experience them as the clients do. It is only when people suspend judgment that they can be free to take on the perspective of the other.

Factors Modulating Empathy

Research has shown that empathy can be modulated voluntarily depending on the intensity of the pain, the affective link between the empathizer and the target, and whether the pain inflicted was seen as a justifiable cure or not (de Vignemont & Singer, 2006). These factors are important to consider in therapy. De Vignemont and Singer (2006) suggest that it may be easier to feel empathy for primary emotions like fear and sadness than for second-ary emotions like jealousy. This supports the view of experiential therapists who actively work to shift clients from states of expressing secondary emotion to the experience and expression of primary emotion. Experiential therapists recognize that it is easier for clients and their partners to respond empathically to primary emotions than to secondary emo-tions. Similarly it may be easier for therapists to respond empathically to clients' primary emotions than to their secondary emotions. Thus therapists' empathic capacity could be enhanced if they are able to help clients shift from expressing secondary emotions to primary emotions. In fact, experiential therapists might use their own level of empathy regarding their clients' experiences to help them discriminate between secondary and primary emotions in their clients.

Second, the relationship between the empathizer and the target of empathy is very impor-tant in determining whether someone will empathize with another. De Vignemont and Singer (2006) suggest a number of factors that may modulate empathy including the simi-larity and familiarity of the target to the empathizer, whether the target is perceived to need nurturance, protection, and care, and whether the emotion is expressed toward the empathizer or somebody else. Rogers (1959) emphasized the importance of therapists' positive regard for their clients. Positive regard was seen as an essential component for building an empathic healing relationship. Thus, therapists have to work at maintaining positive feelings for their clients so as to guard against the loss of empathic capacity as a function of negative feelings. Psychoanalysts have paid a lot of attention to the role of countertransference in therapy, seeing it as both potentially useful and as an impediment to treatment outcomes (Gelso & Hayes, 2001; Richards, 1990). The research from neurosci-ence highlights how important it is for therapists to be aware of the factors that moderate empathy so as to mitigate the effects of negative feelings on their capacity to empathize fully with their clients' experiences.

Another important influence upon empathy consists of the characteristics of the empa-thizer. Rankin and colleagues (2006) distinguished between the cognitive and emotional components of empathy. The cognitive capacities related to empathy include perspective taking, abstract reasoning, and cognitive flexibility. The term *perspective taking* suggests that individuals need to be able to adopt the perspective of others, or to develop a theory of mind by imagining the cognitive and/or emotional state of another based on visual, auditory, or situational cues. *Abstract reasoning* requires that people be able to make interpretations and engage in higher-order reasoning about other people's perspectives, motivations, or intentions. The third cognitive component, *cognitive flexibility*, is differentiated into *spontaneous flexibility* and *reactive flexibility*. Spontaneous flexibility refers to an individual's verbal fluency or ability to quickly and easily generate ideas about another's cognitive and emotional state. Reactive flexibility is the ability of individuals to shift attention back and forth, comparing and contrasting information about their own emotional and cognitive states and those of others in order to sort through various hypotheses and rapidly update working models of other peoples' emotional and cognitive states. The emotional components of empathy include the ability to recognize other peoples' emotions; emotional responsiveness; and the ability to correctly identify one's own emotional and cognitive states.

Some of these characteristics would appear to be innate, and others might be enhanced by training and self-reflection. It is likely that people have different levels of these abilities. Some may be better at the cognitive aspects of empathy whereas others may be more skilled at the emotional components. Ideally, empathic therapists would have the capacities for both the cognitive and affective aspects of empathy. However, it is likely that these skills can be improved. Novice therapists can be taught to read affect more accurately and to be more attentive to affective cues. They can be encouraged to engage in self-reflection in order to increase their level of self-awareness and insight so that they can better differentiate their own feelings from those of their clients. Therapists can be trained to effectively regulate their own emotions so that they do not suffer undue distress or emotional contagion when they work with clients who are experiencing a lot of pain. Cognitive skills can be fostered if novice therapists are encouraged to decenter and to look at problems from multiple perspectives and in different ways.

The complex of characteristics that make up empathy suggests that we can differentiate between cognitive empathy, emotional empathy, and cognitive-emotional empathy. Cognitive empathy may involve different neural systems including mirror motor neurons and the systems that enable perspective taking. It is a form of empathic understanding that is independent of emotional neural networks. Emotional empathy, on the other hand, is based in emotional neural circuits. It is activated by other people's expression of emotion and is founded on one's own understanding of specific situations that might stimulate various emotional responses. A combination of emotional and cognitive aspects of empathy yields the most comprehensive form of empathic understanding, combining a grasp of the other's perspective, and of what things mean to the other, with an understanding of the emotional significance of events.

Although all forms of empathy are expressed in psychotherapy, it is the combination of cognitive and emotional empathy that emotion-focused therapists try to employ to facilitate changes in their clients' ways of being. It is empathy that not only understands the client at a meta level, in terms of what drives them and why they act as they do, but also tries to track clients' moment-to-moment experiences in the session so as to stay responsively attuned to clients as they process their experience. In this way, experiential therapists work to help clients process their affective experience and acquire understanding of why they act as they do, so they can learn new ways of processing their emotions, treating themselves, and interacting with others.

Conclusion

Empathy is a highly complex process that is more than just an epiphenomenon or a background condition of psychotherapy. Empathic understanding integrates information from multiple sources to identify the idiosyncratic meaning of experience for different individuals. Empathic communication results from myriad processes occurring in the brain. It is a synthesis of complex information processing at multiple levels that facilitates human interaction and survival. Empathy is essential to interpersonal communication in every relationship and is a highly sophisticated skill that, when applied or used in the context of psychotherapy, can be very healing. Once we develop an understanding of empathic resonance, it will be important to explore how the communication and receipt of empathy fosters changes in clients' physiology and neurology.

References

Barrett-Lennard, G. T. (1993). The phases and focus of empathy. *British Journal of Medical Psychology, 66*, 3–14.

Barrett-Lennard, G. T. (1997). The recovery of empathy: Toward others and self. In A. C. Bohart & L. S. Greenberg (Eds.), *Empathy reconsidered: New directions in psychotherapy* (pp. 103–121). Washington, DC: American Psychological Association.

Bohart, A. & Greenberg, L. S. (1997). *Empathy reconsidered: New directions in psychotherapy* (pp. 3–31). Washington, DC: American Psychological Association.

Bozarth, J.D. (1997). Empathy from the framework of client-centered theory and the Rogerian hypothesis. In A. Bohart & L. S. Greenberg (Eds.), *Empathy reconsidered: New directions in psychotherapy* (pp. 81–102). Washington, DC: American Psychological Association.

Bucci, W. (1984). Linking words and things: Basic processes and individual variation. *Cognition, 17*, 137–153.

Burns, D. D., & Nolen-Hoeksema, S. (1992). Therapeutic empathy and recovery from depression in cognitive-behavioral therapy: A structural equation model. *Journal of Consulting and Clinical Psychology, 60*, 441–449.

Damasio, A. (1994). *Descartes' error: Emotion, reason, and the human brain*. New York: Putnam.

Danziger, N., Prkachin, K. M., & Willer, J. C. (2006). Is pain the price of empathy? The perception of others' pain in patients with congenital insensitivity to pain. *Brain, 129*, 2494–2507.

Decety, J., & Jackson, P. L. (2004). The functional architecture of human empathy. *Behavioral and Cognitive Neuroscience Reviews, 3*, 71–100.

De Vignemont, F., & Singer, T. (2006). Empathic brain: How, when and why? *Trends in Cognitive Sciences, 10*, 35–41.

Elliott, R., Watson, J. C., Goldman, R. N., & Greenberg, L. S. (2003). Learning emotion-focused therapy: The process-experiential approach to change. Washington, DC: American Psychological Association.

Ferrari, P. F., Gallese, V., Rizzolatti, G., & Fogassi, L. (2003). Mirror neurons responding to the observation of ingestive and communicative mouth actions in the monkey premotor cortex. *European Journal of Neuroscience, 17*, 1703–1714.

Fosha, D. (2001). The dyadic regulation of affect. *Journal of Clinical Psychology, 57*, 227–242.

Gallese, V. (2005). "Being like me": Self-other identity, mirror neurons, and empathy. In S. Hurley & N. Chater (Eds.), *Perspectives on imitation: From neuroscience to social science: Vol. 1. Mechanisms of imitation and imitation in animals* (pp. 101–118). Cambridge, MA: MIT Press.

Gazzola, V., Aziz-Zadeh, L., & Keysers, C. (2006). Empathy and the somatotopic auditory mirror system in humans. *Current Biology, 16*, 1824–1829.

Gelso, C. J., & Hayes, J. A. (2001). Countertransference management. *Psychotherapy, 38* (4), 418–422.

Greenberg, L. S., Rice, L. N., & Elliott, R. (1993). *Facilitating emotional change: The moment-by-moment process.* New York: Guilford Press.

Greenberg, L. S., & Rushanski-Rosenberg, R. (2002). Therapist's experience of empathy. In J. C. Watson, R. N. Goldman, & M. S. Warner (Eds.), *Client-centered and experiential psychotherapy in the 21st century: Advances in theory, research and practice* (168–181). Ross-on Wye, UK: PCCS Books.

Greenberg, L. S., & Watson, J. C. (2006). *Emotionally focused therapy for depression.* Washington, DC: American Psychological Association.

Iacoboni, M., Molnar-Szakacs, I., Gallese, V., Buccino, G., Mazziotta, J. C., & Rizzolatti, G. (2005). Grasping the intentions of others with one's own mirror neuron system. *PLoS Biology, 3*, 529–536.

Jackson, P. L., Brunet, E., Meltzoff, A. N., & Decety, J. (2006). Empathy examined through the neural mechanisms involved imagining how I feel versus how you feel pain. *Neuropsychologia, 44*, 752–761.

Jackson, P. L., & Decety, J. (2004). Motor cognition: A new paradigm to study self-other interactions. *Current Opinion in Neurobiology, 14*, 259–263.

Jackson, P. L., Meltzoff, A. N., & Decety, J. (2005). How do we perceive the pain of others? A window into the neural processes involved in empathy. *NeuroImage, 24*, 771–779.

Kennedy-Moore, E., & Watson, J. C. (1999). *Expressing emotion: Myths, realities and therapeutic strategies.* New York: Guilford Press.

Khan, E. (2002). Heinz Kohut's empathy. In J. C. Watson, R. N. Goldman, & M. S. Warner (Eds.), *Client-centered and experiential psychotherapy in the 21st century: Advances in theory, research, and practice* (pp. 99–104). Ross-on-Wye, UK: PCCS Books.

Klein, M. H., Mathieu-Coughlan, P. L., & Kiesler, D. J. (1986). The Experiencing Scales. In L. S. Greenberg & W. M. Pinsof (Eds.), *The psychotherapeutic process: A research handbook* (pp. 21–71). New York: Guilford Press.

Kohut, H. (1977). *The restoration of self.* New York: International University Press.

Meltzoff, A. N., & Decety, J. (2003). What imitation tells us about social cognition: A rapprochement between developmental psychology and cognitive neuroscience. *Philosophical Transactions of the Royal Society, London, B, 358,* 491–500.

Morrison, I., Lloyd, D., di Pellegrino, G., & Roberts, N. (2004). Vicarious responses to pain in anterior cingulated cortex: Is empathy a multisensory issue? *Cognitive, Affective, & Behavioral Neuroscience, 4,* 270–278.

Preston, S. D., & de Waal, F. B. M. (2002). Empathy: Its ultimate and proximate bases. *Behavioral and Brain Sciences, 25,* 1–72.

Rankin, K. P., Gorno-Tempini, M. L., Allison, S. C., Stanley, C. M., Glenn, S., Weiner, M. W., & Miller, B. L. (2006). Structural anatomy of empathy in neurodegenerative disease. *Brain, 129,* 2945–2956.

Rice, L. N., & Saperia, E. (1984). Task analysis and the resolution of problematic reactions. In L. N. Rice & L. S. Greenberg (Eds.), *Patterns of change: Intensive analysis of psychotherapy process.* New York: Guilford Press.

Richards, J. (1990). Countertransference as a complex tool for understanding the patient in psychotherapy. *Psychoanalytic Psychotherapy, 4* (3), 233–244.

Rizzolatti, G. (2005). The mirror neuron system and imitation. In S. Hurley & N. Chater (Eds.), *Perspectives on imitation: From neuroscience to social science: Vol. 1. Mechanisms of imitation and imitation in animals* (pp. 55–76). Cambridge, MA: MIT Press.

Rogers, C. R. (1951). *Client-centered therapy.* Boston: Houghton-Mifflin.

Rogers, C. R. (1959). A theory of therapy, personality, and interpersonal relationships, as developed in the client-centered framework. In S. Koch (Ed.), *Psychology: The study of a science* (Vol. 3, pp. 184–256). New York: McGraw-Hill.

Rogers, C. R. (1965). *Client-centered therapy: Its current practice, implications and theory.* Boston: Houghton-Mifflin.

Rogers, C. R. (1975). Empathic: An unappreciated way of being. *Counseling Psychologist, 5,* 2–10.

Singer, T., Seymour, B., O'Doherty, J. P. Stephen, K. E., Dolan, R. J., & Frith, C. D. (2006). Empathic neural responses are modulated by the perceived fairness of others. *Nature, 439,* 465–469.

Singer, T., Seymour, B., O'Doherty, J., Kaube, H., Dolan, R. J., & Frith, C. D. (2004). Empathy for pain involves the affective but not sensory components of pain. *Science, 303*, 1157–1162.

Vanaerschot, G. (1990). The process of empathy: Holding and letting go. In G. Lietaer, J. Rombauts, & R. Van Balen (Eds.), *Client-centered and experiential psychotherapy in the nineties* (pp. 269–294). Leuven, Belgium: Leuven University Press.

Warner, M. S. (1997). Does empathy cure? A theoretical consideration of empathy, processing, and personal narrative. In A. C. Bohart & L. S. Greenberg (Eds.), *Empathy reconsidered: New directions in psychotherapy* (pp. 125–140). Washington, DC: American Psychological Association.

Watson, J. C., Goldman, R. N., & Greenberg, L. S. (2007). *Case studies in the emotion focused treatment of depression: A comparison of good and poor outcome.* New York: American Psychological Association.

Watson, J. C. (2001). Revisioning empathy: Theory, research and practice. In D. Cain & J. Seeman (Eds.), *Handbook of research and practice in humanistic psychotherapy* (pp. 445–472). New York: American Psychological Association.

Watson, J. C., & Bohart, A. (2001). Integrative humanistic therapy in an era of managed care. In K. Schneider, J. F. T. Bugenthal, & F. Pierson (Eds.), *The handbook of humanistic psychology* (pp. 503–520). Newbury Park: Sage Publications

Watson, J. C., Goldman, R., & Vanaerschot, G. (1998). Empathic: A postmodern way of being. In L. S. Greenberg, J. C. Watson, & G. Lietaer (Eds.), *Handbook of experiential psychotherapy* (pp. 61–81). New York: Guilford Press.

Watson, J. C., & Greenberg, L. S. (1996). Emotion and cognition in experiential therapy: A dialectical-constructivist position. In H. Rosen & K. Kuelwein (Eds.), *Constructing realities: Meaning-making perspectives for psychotherapists* (pp. 253–276). San Francisco: Jossey-Bass.

Watson, J. C., & Rennie, D. (1994). A qualitative analysis of clients' reports of their subjective experience while exploring problematic reactions in therapy. *Journal of Counseling Psychology, 41*, 500–509.

Wilson, M., & Knoblich, G. (2005). The case for motor involvement in perceiving conspecifics. *Psychological Bulletin, 131*, 460–473.

11 Empathy, Morality, and Social Convention: Evidence from the Study of Psychopathy and Other Psychiatric Disorders

R. J. R. Blair and Karina S. Blair

An association between empathy and moral development has been considered likely for some time (e.g., Hoffman, 1970). However, the nature of the association and the constructs of empathy and moral reasoning themselves have typically been defined rather loosely. The goal of this chapter is to delineate, within the current literature, the relationships between specific neurocognitive systems, the specific forms of empathy they mediate, and specific forms of social-rule-appropriate behavior.

We consider first the nature of empathy and the difference between moral and conventional transgressions. We then consider the role of different forms of emotional empathic response in the emergence of moral and conventional reasoning and how this reasoning is modulated by information regarding the mental states of the transgressors (i.e., cognitive empathy). We conclude by considering responses to other individuals' displays of guilt, shame, and embarrassment following their commission of moral or conventional transgressions.

Defining Empathy

The term *empathy* has been applied to processes enabling the use by the observer of information about the internal state of the observed. There are at least three classes of processing, at least partially separable at both the neural and cognitive levels, that can be described as empathy (Blair, 2005). According to this view, these are *emotional, cognitive* (also known as theory of mind), and *motor* empathy (where the body postures of others mimic those of the observed individual). There are no current data relating motor empathy to moral or social rule development, so only emotional and cognitive empathy will be considered in this chapter.

Emotional Empathy

Emotional responding has been defined as the brain's response to rewarding and punishing stimuli, that is, unconditioned and conditioned appetitive and aversive stimuli (Rolls, 1999). Emotional expressions can be considered reinforcers that have specific communicative functions, imparting specific information to the observer (Blair, 2005). From this view, emotional empathy is defined as the translation of the communication by the observer.

Considerable research has examined the neurocognitive systems that respond to emotional expressions (for a review of this literature, see Adolphs, 2002). This work addresses three main concerns: first, whether there are subcortical systems that respond to emotional expressions; second, whether there are separable neurocognitive systems involved in the processing of different emotional expressions; and third, whether the response to emotional expressions is automatic or under attentional control.

With respect to the issue of subcortical systems, it has been argued that facial expressions are processed not only from visual cortex to limbic areas via temporal cortex but also subcortically (i.e., from thalamus and into limbic areas, in particular, the amygdala; Adolphs, 2002). The issue remains controversial. However, Vuilleumier and colleagues (2003) observed that the pulvinar and the superior colliculus responded to low-frequency but not high-frequency facial expressions; that is, to coarse-grained but not fine-grained information. In short, there appears to be a subcortical route that transmits coarse-grained information about facial expressions to the amygdala in humans, though it may be limited to fearful expressions (Vuilleumier et al., 2003; Luo et al., 2007). This route transmits information to the amygdala rapidly—in less than 40 milliseconds, as indicated by magnetoencephalography (MEG) (Luo et al., 2007).

There is also considerable controversy regarding whether separable neurocognitive systems process different emotional expressions. Some studies have indicated that all emotional expressions activate a similar neural response (Winston, O'Doherty, & Dolan, 2003; Fitzgerald et al., 2006). However, many other studies have not supported this view (see Blair, 2005). The confusion may be due in part to differences in methodology; those studies finding a unitary response have examined four or more expressions simultaneously and may not have had sufficient power to detect differences given the numbers of participants involved (20 and 12 in the Fitzgerald et al., 2006, and Winston et al., 2003, studies respectively).

If, as I have argued, the facial expressions of emotion are reinforcers that have specific communicatory functions (Blair, 2005), then it is unlikely that a unitary system responds to all expressions. This is so because different brain regions are involved in responding to different types of reinforcer. For example, the amygdala is critical for fear-based conditioning (LeDoux, 2000). It is thus unsurprising that fearful expressions preferentially activate the amygdala: one role of fearful expressions may be to rapidly convey information to others that a novel stimulus is aversive and should be avoided (Mineka & Cook, 1993).

The insula, similarly, is critical for taste aversion learning, in addition to its other roles in emotional processing. It is thus unsurprising that disgusted expressions preferentially activate the insula (see Blair, 2005). Disgusted expressions are reinforcers that most frequently provide valence information about foods (for an extended version of this argument, see Blair, 2005).

The response to angry facial expressions seems to represent a second form of empathy. Angry expressions are used to curtail the behavior of others when social rules or expectations have been violated (Averill, 1982). They appear to serve to inform the observer to stop the current behavioral action; they don't necessarily convey any information as to whether that action should be initiated in the future. In other words, angry expressions can be seen as triggers that initiate the reversal of responses (see Blair, 2005). Ventrolateral prefrontal cortex is important for response reversal (Budhani et al., 2007); and, interestingly, similar areas of lateral orbital frontal cortex are activated by angry expressions and by response reversal as a function of contingency change (see Blair, 2005).

With respect to the issue of whether the response to emotional expressions is automatic or under attentional control, there is also a degree of controversy. One view holds that the processing of emotional expressions is "automatic"; the amygdala will show activity in response to fearful expressions whatever the availability of attentional resources (Vuilleumier et al., 2001). The second view suggests that the processing of emotional expressions, like that of neutral stimuli, requires the availability of attentional resources (Pessoa, Padmala, & Morland, 2005). Early findings supported the "automatic" view, pointing to significant amygdala activation in response to unattended stimuli (Vuilleumier et al., 2001). However, these results were surprising. They suggested either that complete amygdala activation could be achieved via the subcortical route (where a case for a lack of attentional modulation can more easily be made) or that, for some reason, emotional stimuli were a class of stimuli for which the principles of representational competition did not apply. According to model of attention developed by Desimone and Duncan (1995), what an individual attends to is the result of a process of competition for neural representation. If the automatic view is correct, it would suggest that the representations of other stimuli could not compete, or interfere, with those of emotional expressions. However, consistent with the view that emotional expressions do compete for representation, later work has shown that manipulations of attention significantly affect the emotional response to both facial expressions and other emotional stimuli (Pessoa, Padmala, & Morland, 2005).

Cognitive Empathy (Theory of Mind)

Cognitive empathy refers to the process by which an individual represents the internal mental state of another individual. This is also the definition of theory of mind (Premack & Woodruff, 1978). Theory of mind allows the attribution of mental states to self and others. At the neural level, research using functional magnetic resonance imaging (fMRI) has implicated the medial prefrontal cortex (especially anterior paracingulate cortex), the temporoparietal junction, and the temporal poles in this ability (for a review, see Frith & Frith, 2006).

Morality versus Social Convention

The previous section considered emotional empathy and argued that emotional expressions are reinforcers that initiate specific types of emotional learning. One form of social interaction that prompts considerable emotional displays and consequent learning is social rule breaking. Moreover, the form of the emotional reactions and the corresponding empathic responses to them by observers in the vicinity differs according to the type of rule transgression committed (Nucci & Turiel, 1978). In this section we briefly consider an important distinction between two types of rule transgression: moral and conventional.

Moral transgressions (e.g., murder and theft) have been defined by their consequences for the rights and welfare of others. In contrast, social convention transgressions (e.g., talking in class or dressing in opposite-gender clothing) have been defined as violations of the behavioral uniformities that structure social interactions within social systems (Turiel, Killen, & Helwig, 1987).

Healthy individuals distinguish moral and conventional transgressions from the age of 39 months (Smetana, 1981) and across cultures (Song, Smetana, & Kim, 1987). They do so in three main ways. First, children and adults usually judge moral transgressions as more serious than conventional transgressions. Second, moral transgressions are judged in a different way than are conventional transgressions. For example, moral transgressions are judged to be less *rule contingent* than conventional transgressions. That is, individuals are less likely to state that moral, rather than conventional, transgressions are permissible in the absence of prohibiting rules. Third, individuals justify the wrongness of moral and conventional transgressions differently. When asked why it is wrong to hit someone or damage their property, participants are significantly more likely to make reference to the suffering of a victim (Smetana, 1981; Song, Smetana, & Kim, 1987; Turiel, Killen, & Helwig, 1987). In contrast, when asked why it is wrong to talk in class or wear opposite-gender clothes (conventional transgressions), participants will make reference to established rules that can be either explicit (that action is prohibited in this school) or implicit (that action is "not the done thing").

It is the presence or absence of victims that distinguishes moral from conventional transgressions (Smetana, 1985). If a participant believes that a transgression will result in a victim, she or he will process that transgression as moral. If a participant believes that a transgression will not result in a victim, s/he will process that transgression as conventional. For example, Smetana (1985) found that unknown transgressions (specified by a nonsense word; e.g., X has done dool) were processed as moral or conventional according to the specified consequences of the act. Thus, "X has done dool and made Y cry" would be processed as moral whereas "X has done dool and the teacher told him off" would be processed as conventional.

Emotional Empathy and Moral and Conventional Reasoning

As noted above, the socioemotional consequences of moral and conventional transgressions differ. Specifically, adults respond differentially to them. Moral transgressions can be associated with the distress (fear, sadness) of the victim and are more likely to elicit empathy induction by caregivers. Conventional transgressions are more likely to result in power-assertive expressions or behaviors by caregivers, such as anger (Nucci & Turiel, 1978). The argument to be developed here is that these differing socioemotional consequences are the causal origins of the child's distinction between moral and conventional transgressions.

Moral Reasoning and Emotional Empathic Responses to Victims

We have posited that fearful and sad expressions have the effect of rapidly conveying information to others that the stimuli associated with these expressions should be avoided. By this account, moral socialization involves associating the victim's distress with the action that caused the distress. Empathy induction techniques, shown to be particularly effective in moral socialization (Hoffman, 1970), should work because they focus the individual's attention on the distress of the victim. As shown above, increasing the attention focused on an emotional stimulus should increase the emotional response to that stimulus (Pessoa et al., 2002). This view predicts that a population who are significantly less emotionally responsive to the distress of others should show difficulties in moral socialization. We will argue that individuals with psychopathy represent such a population.

Psychopathy is a disorder characterized in part by callousness—that is, a diminished capacity for remorse—impulsivity, and poor behavioral control (Hare, 1991). The disorder involves two core components: emotional dysfunction (reduced guilt, empathy, and attachment to significant others) and antisocial behavior (Hare, 1991). It is a developmental disorder that appears in childhood and extends throughout the life span (Harpur & Hare, 1994).

Individuals with psychopathy show clear impairment in processing the fearfulness and sadness of others. Thus, children and adults with psychopathy typically show impairment in the recognition of fearful and, to a lesser extent, sad facial (Blair et al., 2001) and vocal expressions (Blair et al., 2002). Moreover, they show reduced autonomic responses to the distress of others (Blair et al., 1997) and reduced attentional biases to the distress of others (Kimonis et al., 2006).

In line with the argument that an appropriate emotional response—that is, an empathic response—to the distress of others is crucial for moral socialization, children and adults with psychopathy show significantly less of a differentiation between moral and conventional transgressions on the moral-conventional distinction task (Blair, 1995). They also fail to show appropriate associations of negative affect with moral transgressions when these are examined using morality implicit association task paradigms (Gray et al., 2003). Such paradigms require the participant to make the same response to either congruently valenced (i.e., respond left to immoral items and nasty animals) or incongruently valenced (i.e., respond left to immoral items and nice animals) response options. The degree of interference (slower RTs) when using the same response option for incongruently valenced rather than congruently valenced response options is thought to index the individual's level implicit association of the item groups. Other research has shown that individuals who show high levels of the emotion dysfunction associated with psychopathy are less responsive to socialization techniques. Thus it appears that the emotion dysfunction directly interferes with moral socialization (Wootton et al., 1997).

According to the argument developed here, the important empathic process with respect to moral socialization is the translation of the victim's distress such that stimulus-reinforcement learning occurs; the victim's distress is aversive to the healthy individual, who learns to avoid the action that has caused the other harm. As argued above, the amygdala is very important in stimulus-reinforcement learning (LeDoux, 2000). Considerable data suggest amygdala dysfunction in psychopathy (for a review, see Blair, Mitchell, & Blair, 2005). For example, individuals with psychopathy show impairment in aversive conditioning (Flor et al., 2002), an important function of the amygdala (LeDoux, 1998), and, indeed, reduced amygdala activity during aversive conditioning (Birbaumer et al., 2005) and other forms of emotional learning (Kiehl et al., 2001). Moreover, individuals with psychopathy show impairment in stimulus-reinforcement based instrumental learning tasks (Blair, Leonard, et al., 2006). Such tasks require the functional integrity of the amygdala (Blair, Marsh, et al., 2006).

The amygdala has considerable reciprocal interconnection with medial frontal cortex (Amaral et al., 1992). It can be argued that the amygdala, following stimulus-reinforcement learning, feeds forward reinforcement-expectancy information to the medial frontal cortex (Blair, 2004). The medial frontal cortex allows the representation of this reinforcement information, predisposing the individual to either approach or avoid the object or action (Blair, Marsh, et al., 2006).

Recent neuroimaging studies of morality using a diverse range of methodologies, including a morality implicit association task, have implicated both the amygdala and medial regions of orbital frontal cortex (Greene et al., 2001; Luo et al., 2006). We argue that the amygdala plays a role in morality by allowing the association of representation of transgressions (interpersonal violence) with the victim's fear or sadness (Blair, 1995). We believe that medial orbital frontal cortical activation allows the representation of reinforcement expectations (information provided by the amygdala), and that this information guides the individual's tendency to approach or avoid the object or action (Blair, 2004). In short, the information allows the individual to engage in moral decision making; the integrated response of the amygdala and the orbital frontal cortex is the neural basis of the individual's "moral intuition."

Although the account developed above describes the emotional response to a moral transgression and how this response would guide behavior away from such a transgression (and also generate negative attitudes toward it), it does not discriminate between a victim's distress caused by a natural disaster or by a human agent. In short, the system described would set up an aversive attitude to both a natural disaster and a human agent causing harm to others. Such a system might therefore allow judgments of "badness" but not judgments of immorality (cf. Nichols, 2002). To understand judgments of immorality, we need to consider cognitive empathy, and the next section examines the relationship between cognitive empathy and moral reasoning. First, however, we briefly consider social convention.

Emotional Empathic Responses to Another's Anger and Reasoning about Conventions

At one time it was argued that morality could be distinguished from convention because only morality was associated with emotional responses (Kagan & Lamb, 1987). However, there are clear emotional responses associated with conventional transgressions. For example, the teacher experiencing a child continuously talking in the classroom is likely to feel anger. In short, moral and conventional transgressions cannot be distinguished on grounds that only the former elicit emotional responses. However, moral and conventional transgressions *can* be distinguished because they are associated with *different* emotional responses.

We suggested above that a distinct form of empathy involves the response to angry expressions. We argued, following Averill (1982), that angry expressions curtail the behavior of others when social rules or expectations have been violated; they inform their intended recipient to stop the current behavioral action or face the consequences. We have also noted research supporting the notion that angry expressions initiate this modification of behavior through the recruitment of the ventrolateral prefrontal cortex (see Blair, 2005).

Conventional transgressions are considered to be bad because of their disruption of the social order (Turiel et al., 1987). Societal rules concerning conventional transgressions function to allow higher-status individuals to constrain the behavior of lower-status individuals. By their operation they may also serve to reduce within-species conflict by reinforcing hierarchies. Indeed, it has been suggested that the human angry expression evolved to mimic a high-status, dominant face (Marsh, Adams, & Kleck, 2005). Moreover, high-status nonverbal cues activate the regions that also respond to angry expressions and other cues for behavioral modification; specifically, the ventrolateral prefrontal cortex.

We argue that aversive social cues (particularly—but not only—angry expressions) or expectations of such cues activate ventrolateral prefrontal cortex. (Expectations of aversive social cues would be engendered by representations previously associated with the aversive cues, e.g., representations of actions that make other individuals angry.) This ventrolateral prefrontal cortex activation (1) guides the individual away from committing conventional transgressions (particularly in the presence of higher-status individuals) and (2) orchestrates a response to witnessed conventional transgressions (particularly when they are committed by lower-status individuals), such as submission or becoming angry in turn (see Blair, 2005). In short, reasoning about social conventions should and does activate ventrolateral prefrontal cortex (Berthoz et al., 2002).

This position predicts that individuals with impairment to ventrolateral prefrontal cortex will show impairment when reasoning about conventional transgressions. Two patient populations are of clear relevance to this prediction. The first are neurological patients with lesions of orbital and/or ventrolateral frontal cortex. Such patients exhibit difficulties with expression recognition (Blair & Cipolotti, 2000). In line with the prediction, patients with such lesions also show difficulties processing conventional transgressions, as indexed by performance on tasks requiring appropriate responses to such transgressions (see Blair & Cipolotti, 2000).

The second population is children with bipolar disorder. Childhood bipolar disorder is marked by emotional lability and irritability (Leibenluft et al., 2003). Neuropsychological and neuroimaging data suggest that at least part of the pathology seen in these children is related to ventrolateral prefrontal cortex dysfunction (Gorrindo et al., 2005). In addition, children with bipolar disorder show impairment in expression recognition (McClure et al., 2003) and on social cognition tasks where the processing of conventional rules is important (McClure et al., 2005).

Cognitive Empathy and Moral and Conventional Reasoning

At one time, it was assumed that emotional empathic responses required the ability to represent the mental states of others (Feshbach, 1978). This view suggests that a population with impairment in the ability to represent the mental states of others (a population lacking theory of mind) should show impaired empathy and, by inference, moral reasoning.

Autism is a severe developmental disorder described by the American Psychiatric Association's diagnostic and statistical manual (*DSM-IV*) as "the presence of markedly abnormal or impaired development in social interaction and communication and a markedly restricted repertoire of activities and interests" (American Psychiatric Association, 1994, p. 66). The main criteria for the diagnosis of autism in the *DSM-IV* can be summarized as qualitative impairment in social communication and restricted and repetitive patterns of behavior and interests.

Considerable data suggest that individuals with autism are impaired in the representation of the mental states of others (see, for a review, Hill & Frith, 2003). Moreover, neuroimaging has revealed reduced activation in individuals with autism spectrum disorders in those brain regions critical to the representation of the mental states of others (i.e., medial prefrontal cortex, temporoparietal junction, and the temporal poles; Castelli et al., 2002).

With respect to the issue of emotional empathy in autism, there is some confusion in the literature. Older work consistently reported that individuals with autism have difficulty recognizing the emotional expressions of others (e.g., Hobson, 1986). However, these studies were criticized because they did not match groups for mental age. When this is done, group differences often disappear (Adolphs, Sears, & Pivens, 2001), but not always (Humphreys et al., 2007). There is also evidence that children with autism show autonomic responses to the distress of others (Blair, 1999) and that at least those who are more cognitively able are appropriately emotionally responsive to the distress of others (Corona et al., 1998). In short, there are reasons to believe that the basic emotional empathic response—that is, the engagement of emotional learning systems following the presentation of emotional expression—is intact in individuals with autism. Consistent with this view, individuals with autism appear to have basic moral intuitions: they show no significant impairment on the moral-conventional distinction test (Blair, 1996).

But this does not mean that theory of mind is irrelevant to moral reasoning. Beginning with Piaget, a considerable research literature has accumulated that points to the importance of information about the perpetrator's intent when people assign moral blame or praise (Piaget, 1932). It is this information that allows us to decide that an action is immoral rather than just a bad thing to have occurred. The person who intentionally swings a baseball bat into someone else's face has behaved far more "immorally" than the individual who accidentally swings a baseball bat into another person's face. In line with suggestions that theory of mind is necessary for the integration of information about intention into moral reasoning, individuals with autism show reduced integration of such information into their moral reasoning (Steele, Joseph, & Tager-Flusberg, 2003).

In short, actions that are "wrong" rather than merely "bad" are acts where there is intent to cause harm. The actions of an intentional agent that cause harm to others are wrong. The actions of an unintentional agent (including natural disasters unless these are attributed to a divine intent) are just bad. As the level of victim distress increases, the act comes to be regarded as more "wrong" or more "bad" depending on the intention associated with the action. As it becomes clearer that the intent of the transgressor was to cause harm, the act becomes progressively more likely to be regarded as wrong rather than bad. Similarly, information about the mental states of others can modulate the response to apparent transgressors of social conventions. Someone who purposely takes another person's seat on a train causes considerably greater irritation than a person who accidentally falls into another person's seat on the train.

Empathic Responses to Appeasement Displays

Various authors have suggested that guilt, shame, and embarrassment serve an important social function by signaling appeasement and the desire to make restitution to others (Keltner & Buswell, 1997). When a person's untoward behavior threatens his or her standing in an important social group, visible signs of guilt, shame, or embarrassment function as a nonverbal acknowledgment of shared social standards. The specific emotion displayed is partly a function of the transgression. Whereas moral transgressions are associated with guilt, shame, and embarrassment, conventional transgressions are associated only with embarrassment and shame (Finger et al., 2006). Considerable empirical evidence from studies of both humans and nonhuman primates supports the "appeasement" or remedial function of these social emotions (Keltner & Buswell, 1997).

If the social emotions serve an important social function by signaling appeasement, the individual's perceived intention is likely to be crucial in determining whether they are displayed. If someone *intends* to transgress, we might suspect that the person will not display guilt or shame or embarrassment afterward. If the transgression is intentional the transgressor is unlikely to be interested in the social relationship that has been broken. In contrast, if the violation of the social convention was unintended, we might expect clear displays of appeasement-related emotion according to the nature of the transgression; the person recognizes the transgression and wishes to restore the social relationship. Research on embarrassment at least suggests that this is the case (Berthoz et al., 2002).

Seeing or hearing about another person committing a moral or conventional transgression, or committing such a transgression oneself, should lead to response modulation and associated ventrolateral prefrontal cortex activation. The desire to prompt appeasement or restitution acts from another person, or to engage in these acts oneself, should compete with motor responses engaged by current task demands. The existing data are consistent with this claim (Berthoz et al., 2002; Finger et al., 2006). It can be predicted, though this is currently untested, that displays of appeasement or restitution by the transgressors should reduce this brain activity. However, it is known that the presence or absence of an audience while committing transgressions has an impact on ventrolateral prefrontal cortex activity and that the impact is transgression specific (Finger et al., 2006). Moral transgressions in healthy individuals should initiate appeasement/restitution behaviors whether or not an audience is present because the victim has been hurt. Conventional transgressions should initiate such behaviors only if there is an audience. This reasoning predicts that ventrolateral prefrontal cortex activation should occur with moral transgressions whether or not an audience witnesses the action but that conventional transgressions should initiate this activation only if an audience is present. This prediction has recently been confirmed (Finger et al., 2006).

Conclusions

In this chapter we have argued that the association between empathy and morality is not a simple one. Rather, there is an association between different forms of empathic processes and different forms of social rule. Specifically, the empathic response to fearful and sad expressions is associated with the development of proscriptions against moral transgressions, while the empathic response to angry expressions is associated with the development of proscriptions against conventional transgressions. In addition, whereas emotional empathic responses are important for the development of proscriptions against these different forms of social rule, cognitive empathic responses—that is, representations of the other's intent—can have considerable impact on the observer's attitude toward the transgressor. Unintentional transgressions of moral and conventional rules are regarded as significantly less serious than intentional transgressions. Finally, an individual's empathic response to displays of appeasement (guilt, shame, and embarrassment, depending on the transgression type) significantly modulates that individual's attitude toward the transgressor.

References

Adolphs, R. (2002). Neural systems for recognizing emotion. *Current Opinion in Neurobiology, 12* (2), 169–177.

Adolphs, R., Sears, L., & Piven, J. (2001). Abnormal processing of social information from faces in autism. *Journal of Cognitive Neuroscience, 13* (2), 232–240.

Amaral, D. G., Price, J. L., Pitkanen, A., & Carmichael, S. T. (1992). Anatomical organization of the primate amygdaloid complex. In J. P. Aggleton (Ed.), *The amygdala: Neurobiological aspects of emotion, memory, and mental dysfunction* (pp. 1–66). New York: Wiley.

American Psychiatric Association. (1994). *Diagnostic and statistical manual of mental disorders* (4th ed.). Washington, DC: American Psychiatric Association.

Averill, J. R. (1982). *Anger and aggression: An essay on emotion.* New York: Springer.

Berthoz, S., Armony, J., Blair, R. J. R., & Dolan, R. (2002). Neural correlates of violation of social norms and embarrassment. *Brain, 125* (8), 1696–1708.

Birbaumer, N., Veit, R., Lotze, M., Erb, M., Hermann, C., Grodd, W., & Flor, H. (2005). Deficient fear conditioning in psychopathy: A functional magnetic resonance imaging study. *Archives of General Psychiatry, 62* (7), 799–805.

Blair, K. S., Leonard, A., Morton, J. & Blair, R. J. R. (2006). Impaired decision making on the basis of both reward and punishment information in individuals with psychopathy. *Personality and Individual Differences, 41,* 155–165.

Blair, K. S., Marsh, A. A., Morton, J., Vythilingham, M., Jones, M., Mondillo, K., Pine, D. S., Drevets, W. C., & Blair, R. J. R. (2006). Choosing the lesser of two evils, the better of two goods: Specifying the roles of ventromedial prefrontal cortex and dorsal anterior cingulate cortex in object choice. *Journal of Neuroscience, 26* (44), 11379–11386.

Blair, R. J. R. (1995). A cognitive developmental approach to morality: Investigating the psychopath. *Cognition, 57,* 1–29.

Blair, R. J. R. (1996). Brief report: Morality in the autistic child. *Journal of Autism and Developmental Disorders, 26,* 571–579.

Blair, R. J. R. (1999). Psycho-physiological responsiveness to the distress of others in children with autism. *Personality and Individual Differences, 26,* 477–485.

Blair, R. J. R. (2004). The roles of orbital frontal cortex in the modulation of antisocial behavior. *Brain and Cognition, 55* (1), 198–208.

Blair, R. J. R. (2005). Responding to the emotions of others: Dissociating forms of empathy through the study of typical and psychiatric populations. *Consciousness and Cognition, 14* (4), 698–718.

Blair, R. J. R., & Cipolotti, L. (2000). Impaired social response reversal: A case of "acquired sociopathy." *Brain, 123,* 1122–1141.

Blair, R. J. R., Colledge, E., Murray, L., & Mitchell, D. G. (2001). A selective impairment in the processing of sad and fearful expressions in children with psychopathic tendencies. *Journal of Abnormal Child Psychology, 29* (6), 491–498.

Blair, R. J. R., Jones, L., Clark, F., & Smith, M. (1997). The psychopathic individual: A lack of responsiveness to distress cues? *Psychophysiology, 34,* 192–198.

Blair, R. J. R., Mitchell, D. G. V., & Blair, K. S. (2005). *The psychopath: Emotion and the brain.* Oxford: Blackwell.

Blair, R. J. R., Mitchell, D. G. V., Richell, R. A., Kelly, S., Leonard, A., Newman, C., & Scott, S. K. (2002). Turning a deaf ear to fear: Impaired recognition of vocal affect in psychopathic individuals. *Journal of Abnormal Psychology, 111* (4), 682–686.

Budhani, S., Marsh, A. A., Pine, D. S., & Blair, R. J. (2007). Neural correlates of response reversal: Considering acquisition. *NeuroImage, 34* (4), 1754–1765.

Castelli, F., Frith, C., Happe, F., & Frith, U. (2002). Autism, Asperger syndrome and brain mechanisms for the attribution of mental states to animated shapes. *Brain, 125,* 1839–1849.

Corona, C., Dissanayake, C., Arbelle, A., Wellington, P., & Sigman, M. (1998). Is affect aversive to young children with autism? Behavioural and cardiac responses to experimenter distress. *Child Development, 69* (6), 1494–1502.

Desimone, R., & Duncan, J. (1995). Neural mechanisms of selective visual attention. *Annual Review of Neuroscience, 18,* 193–222.

Feshbach, N. D. (1978). Studies of empathic behavior in children. In B. A. Maher (Ed.), *Progress in experimental personality research* (pp. 1–47). New York: Academic Press.

Finger, E. C., Marsh, A. A., Kamel, N., Mitchell, D. G., & Blair, J. R. (2006). Caught in the act: The impact of audience on the neural response to morally and socially inappropriate behavior. *NeuroImage, 33* (1), 414–421.

Fitzgerald, D. A., Angstadt, M., Jelsone, L. M., Nathan, P. J., & Phan, K. L. (2006). Beyond threat: Amygdala reactivity across multiple expressions of facial affect. *NeuroImage, 30* (4), 1441–1448.

Flor, H., Birbaumer, N., Hermann, C., Ziegler, S., & Patrick, C. J. (2002). Aversive Pavlovian conditioning in psychopaths: Peripheral and central correlates. *Psychophysiology 39,* 505–518.

Frith, C. D., & Frith, U. (2006). The neural basis of mentalizing. *Neuron, 50* (4), 531–534.

Gorrindo, T., Blair, R. J., Budhani, S., Dickstein, D. P., Pine, D. S., & Leibenluft, E. (2005). Deficits on a probabilistic response-reversal task in patients with pediatric bipolar disorder. *American Journal of Psychiatry, 162* (10), 1975–1977.

Gray, N. S., MacCulloch, M. J., Smith, J., Morris, M., & Snowden, R. J. (2003). Forensic psychology: Violence viewed by psychopathic murderers. *Nature, 423,* 497–498.

Greene, J. D., Sommerville, R. B., Nystrom, L. E., Darley, J. M., & Cohen, J. D. (2001). An fMRI investigation of emotional engagement in moral judgment. *Science, 293,* 1971–1972.

Hare, R. D. (1991). *The Hare Psychopathy Checklist—Revised*. Toronto: Multi-Health Systems.

Harpur, T. J., & Hare, R. D. (1994). Assessment of psychopathy as a function of age. *Journal of Abnormal Psychology, 103*, 604–609.

Hill, E. L., & Frith, U. (2003). Understanding autism: Insights from mind and brain. *Philosophical Transactions of the Royal Society, London, B, 358* (1430), 281–289.

Hobson, P. (1986). The autistic child's appraisal of expressions of emotion. *Journal of Child Psychology and Psychiatry, 27*, 321–342.

Hoffman, M. L. (1970). Conscience, personality and socialization techniques. *Human Development, 13*, 90–126.

Humphreys, K., Minshew, N., Leonard, G. L., & Behrmann, M. (2007). A fine-grained analysis of facial expression processing in high-functioning adults with autism. *Neuropsychologia, 45* (4), 685–695.

Kagan, J., & Lamb, S. (1987). *The emergence of morality in young children*. Chicago: University of Chicago Press.

Keltner, D., & Buswell, B. N. (1997). Embarrassment: Its distinct form and appeasement functions. *Psychological Bulletin, 122* (3), 250–270.

Kiehl, K. A., Smith, A. M., Hare, R. D., Mendrek, A., Forster, B. B., Brink, J., & Liddle, P. F. (2001). Limbic abnormalities in affective processing by criminal psychopaths as revealed by functional magnetic resonance imaging. *Biological Psychiatry, 50*, 677–684.

Kimonis, E. R., Frick, P. J., Fazekas, H., & Loney, B. R. (2006). Psychopathy, aggression, and the processing of emotional stimuli in non-referred girls and boys. *Behavioral Sciences and the Law, 24* (1), 21–37.

LeDoux, J. E. (1998). *The emotional brain*. New York: Weidenfeld & Nicolson.

LeDoux, J. E. (2000). The amygdala and emotion: A view through fear. In J. P. Aggleton (Ed.), *The amygdala: A functional analysis* (pp. 289–31). Oxford: Oxford University Press.

Leibenluft, E., Blair, R. J., Charney, D. S., & Pine, D. S. (2003). Irritability in pediatric mania and other childhood psychopathology. *Annals of the New York Academy of Sciences, 1008*, 201–218.

Luo, Q., Holroyd, T., Jones, M., Hendler, T., & Blair, J. (2007). Neural dynamics for facial threat processing as revealed by gamma band synchronization using MEG. *NeuroImage, 34* (2), 839–847.

Luo, Q., Nakic, M., Wheatley, T., Richell, R., Martin, A., & Blair, R. J. (2006). The neural basis of implicit moral attitude: An IAT study using event-related fMRI. *NeuroImage, 30* (4), 1449–1457.

Marsh, A. A., Adams, R. B., & Kleck, R. E. (2005). Why do fear and anger look the way they do? Form and social function in facial expressions. *Personality and Social Psychology Bulletin, 31*, 1–14.

McClure, E. B., Pope, K., Hoberman, A. J., Pine, D. S., & Leibenluft, E. (2003). *Facial expression recognition in adolescents with mood and anxiety disorders*. American Journal of Psychiatry, 160 (6), 1172–1174.

McClure, E. B., Treland, J. E., Snow, J., Schmajuk, M., Dickstein, D. P., Towbin, K. E., Charney, D. S., Pine, D. S., & Leibenluft, E. (2005). Deficits in social cognition and response flexibility in pediatric bipolar disorder. *American Journal of Psychiatry, 162* (9), 1644–1651.

Mineka, S., & Cook, M. (1993). Mechanisms involved in the observational conditioning of fear. *Journal of Experimental Psychology: General*, *122*, 23–38.

Nichols, S. (2002). Norms with feeling: Towards a psychological account of moral judgment. *Cognition*, *84* (2), 221–236.

Nucci, L. P., & Turiel, E. (1978). Social interactions and the development of social concepts in preschool children. *Child Development*, *49*, 400–407.

Pessoa, L., McKenna, M., Gutierrez, E., & Ungerleider, L. G. (2002). Neural processing of emotional faces requires attention. *Proceedings of the National Academy of Sciences USA*, *99*, 11458–11463.

Pessoa, L., Padmala, S., & Morland, T. (2005). Fate of unattended fearful faces in the amygdala is determined by both attentional resources and cognitive modulation. *NeuroImage*, *28* (1), 249–255.

Piaget, J. (1932). *The moral development of the child.* London: Routledge & Kegan Paul.

Premack, D., & Woodruff, G. (1978). Does the chimpanzee have a theory of mind? *Behavioral and Brain Sciences*, *1* (4), 515–526.

Rolls, E. T. (1999). *The brain and emotion.* Oxford: Oxford University Press.

Smetana, J. G. (1981). Preschool children's conceptions of moral and social rules. *Child Development*, *52*, 1333–1336.

Smetana, J. G. (1985). Preschool children's conceptions of transgressions: The effects of varying moral and conventional domain-related attributes. *Developmental Psychology*, *21*, 18–29.

Song, M., Smetana, J. G., & Kim, S. Y. (1987). Korean children's conceptions of moral and conventional transgressions. *Developmental Psychology*, *23*, 577–582.

Steele, S., Joseph, R. M., & Tager-Flusberg, H. (2003). Brief report: Developmental change in theory of mind abilities in children with autism. *Journal of Autism and Developmental Disorders*, *33*, 461–467.

Turiel, E., Killen, M., & Helwig, C. C. (1987). Morality: Its structure, functions, and vagaries. In J. Kagan & S. Lamb (Eds.), *The emergence of morality in young children* (pp. 155–245). Chicago: University of Chicago Press.

Vuilleumier, P., Armony, J. L., Driver, J., & Dolan, R. J. (2001). Effects of attention and emotion on face processing in the human brain: An event-related fMRI study. *Neuron*, *30* (3), 829–841.

Vuilleumier, P., Armony, J. L., Driver, J., & Dolan, R. J. (2003). Distinct spatial frequency sensitivities for processing faces and emotional expressions. *Nature Neuroscience*, *6* (6), 624–631.

Winston, J. S., O'Doherty, J., & Dolan, R. J. (2003). Common and distinct neural responses during direct and incidental processing of multiple facial emotions. *NeuroImage*, *20* (1), 84–97.

Wootton, J. M., Frick, P. J., Shelton, K. K., & Silverthorn, P. (1997). Ineffective parenting and childhood conduct problems: The moderating role of callous-unemotional traits. *Journal of Consulting and Clinical Psychology*, *65*, 292–300.

12 Perceiving Others in Pain: Experimental and Clinical Evidence on the Role of Empathy

Liesbet Goubert, Kenneth D. Craig, and Ann Buysse

The complexities of human life often necessitate sensitivity to the behavior of others. Perhaps unsurpassed in importance for both personal and group survival is attention to the experiences of others when they confront physical danger and pain. Knowing other people's feelings, thoughts, and behavioral reactions in the context of what is happening to them may be vital if the observing persons are to protect themselves or deliver care to the other person. When witnessing another person experiencing pain, the scope of observer reactions can range from concern for personal safety, including feelings of alarm and fear, to concern for the other person, including compassion, sympathy, and interest in caregiving, among other possibilities. Although it is recognized that precursors to the capacity for empathy were biologically and behaviorally present and conserved in nonhuman species (e.g., see Preston & de Waal, 2002; Langford et al., 2006), this chapter will review research addressing the nature and the determinants of the *human* observer's empathic reactions and their consequences for both the observer and the suffering person in clinical and everyday life settings.

Definitional Issues

Conceptualizing the nature of empathy for pain requires careful consideration of both concepts. Viewing empathic reactions as multidimensional (Davis, 1996), we have recently proposed that the core of empathy can be understood as a sense of knowing the personal experience of another person (Goubert et al., 2005), a cognitive appreciation that is accompanied by both affective and behavioral responses.

Empathy: A Multidimensional Construct

Having a sense of knowing the other person's thoughts, feelings, and motives can be considered the *cognitive* component of empathy, but the *affective* component of empathic responses is also central to and helps to organize the experience. The cognitive component concerns the extent to which the observer understands the nature of the other person's thoughts and feelings, a topic to be addressed below. There are two main categories of affective empathy responses to observing another person in pain: responses oriented to the self and responses oriented to the other (Goubert et al., 2009). Self-oriented affective responses are feelings of distress and anxiety when witnessing another's negative experiences, whereas responses oriented to the other comprise feelings that focus on the well-being of the other person, including concern or sympathy for that person (Davis, 1996). Although these two types of *affective* responses can occur together, they are qualitatively distinct. They imply different motivational *behavioral* tendencies; respectively, reducing one's own distress versus being oriented to the needs of the other and motivated to engage in caregiving (Batson, 1991). To constitute pain empathy, an observer's self-oriented responses must include at least some element of similarity to the feelings of painful distress experienced by the observed person. One can also conceptualize discordant affective responses to observed pain in others, including pleasure when others are in distress (e.g., schadenfreude, sadistic reactions) or knowledge of the other's plight in the absence of emotional distress (e.g., psychopathic reactions).

The Complexities of Pain

Pain is not a unidimensional experience, as use of the term in common parlance sometimes implies (Williams & Craig, 2006). It encompasses manifold sensory inputs, as well as thoughts and feelings that inevitably are highly individual because they reflect the person's unique life experience. The broad nature of the phenomenon is captured in the following standard definition of pain: "An unpleasant sensory and emotional experience associated with actual or potential tissue damage, or described in terms of such damage" (Merskey & Bogduk, 1994). The complexity of pain therefore poses a major challenge for the observer who wants to know the nature of another person's pain.

Benefits and Limitations of Accurate Empathy

Although "sense of knowing" does not necessarily imply *accurate* knowing, many studies in the domain of interpersonal relationships have examined the congruence between the person's inner experience and the observer's inferences of it (e.g., Ickes, 2001). It is generally assumed that a certain level of accuracy in one's "sense of knowing," and some similarity in one's affective responses, are necessary but not sufficient conditions for prosocial behavior (Charbonneau & Nicol, 2002) and effective caregiving.

With regard to empathy for pain, there are limits to the extent to which the experiences of the person in pain and the observer can be isomorphic (Goubert et al., 2005; Jackson, Rainville, & Decety, 2006). Perception of pain in others is likely to be an incomplete representation of pain in oneself (Jackson, Brunet, et al., 2006). Functional magnetic resonance imaging (fMRI) research has demonstrated that—in contrast to the person who is experiencing pain—only brain regions involved in affective, but not sensory, responding are activated in observers (Singer et al., 2004). In other words, observers lack the somatic input fundamental to the personal experience of pain. Similarly, affective responses (in particular, distress responses) to observing another person in pain would be expected to correspond to the responses of the suffering person with varying degrees of exactness, because the threat of personal harm arises from a different source.

For the individual in pain, self-interest is likely to prevail, and attention is focused on one's own pain sensations, probably accompanied by thoughts and feelings regarding the personal impact of the injury or disease. In observers, however, attention may be focused upon the other's pain expressions, and distress responses might reflect processes of emotional contagion, wherein observers mirror the distress of the other without necessarily having an awareness of the other's internal experience. Although these contagion-like processes are in most situations more or less automatically initiated (conceivably involving mirror-neuron mechanisms; see, e.g., Gallese, Keysers, & Rizzolatti, 2004), they may also be modulated by higher-order cognitive factors, such as the observer's thoughts about the pain that the other is experiencing.

Different strategies have been developed to determine how accurate observers are in their judgments of others' (pain-related) thoughts, feelings, and motives, and to what extent accurate inferences have the potential to yield benefits for the suffering person, the observer, and their relationship. Ickes (2003) showed that accuracy in interpersonal judgments is far from perfect. Using the empathic accuracy methodology, which measures the degree to which the thought-feeling events reported by a target person are accurately inferred by a target's interaction partner (the observer), the data from many studies show that the typical range of mean empathic accuracy scores is from 15% to 35% (W. Ickes, personal communication, February 2, 2005). These numbers suggest that observers have some ability to accurately infer what another person is thinking or feeling, but that they are often relatively unsuccessful. In most social interactions, people are "good enough" perceivers rather than "perfectly accurate" in understanding others' subjective experiences (Fiske, 1993).

In the field of pain research, many studies show discrepancies in pain estimations between persons in pain and observers. Using unidimensional self-report judgments of pain provided by both people in pain and observers, most studies have reported underestimations of pain by observers (Chambers et al., 1998), although some studies have reported overestimation (e.g., Redinbaugh et al., 2002). Common sense suggests that accuracy in pain assessment is essential for effective pain treatment. Indeed, underestimation of pain carries the risk of the person in pain receiving inadequate care and feeling misunderstood, consequences that are potentially devastating to the person in pain. On the other hand, overestimations of pain entail risks such as unnecessary medication or overprotective behavior on the part of observers (Goubert et al., 2005).

It is also important to question whether accuracy in estimating another's pain and substantial similarity in affective responding (e.g., distress) are related to the instigation of effective helping behavior. In professional settings dispassionate concern for the patient is encouraged in the interests of objective care. It would be worthwhile to investigate whether greater similarity in affective responses is associated with more accurate inference of the internal experience of the person in pain, thereby affecting helping behavior (see Levenson & Ruef, 1992).

On the other hand, there may be benefits to maintaining a less than perfect accuracy level by making inferences that are just adequate to enable effective actions (Jussim, 1991). To "max out" on accuracy in knowing what the other is experiencing could incur costly cognitive and affective demands (Hodges & Klein, 2001). It is conceivable that highly accurate observers would be characterized as oversensitive, suffering unduly (Schaller & Cialdini, 1988) and having difficulty in delivering effective helping behavior. High accuracy could fuel a cascade of distress and helplessness in both the observer and the person in pain (see Goubert et al., 2005). Exposure among professionals and volunteers to high levels of pain and suffering can lead to vicarious traumatization, as evidenced by high levels of professional "burnout" in clinical settings where unremitting pain is a serious problem, such as burn units (Palm, Polusny, & Follette, 2004). In some instances, therefore, observers who respond with high distress to the perception of another individual in pain might be motivated to underestimate the observed person's pain, in an attempt to keep their own distress within acceptable limits (Goubert et al., 2005) or to constrain the other's pain-related emotional expression (Herbette & Rimé, 2004).

In summary, it is possible that observers with average empathic accuracy scores, having a general "sense of knowing" the experience of the other in pain, might be the most effective in delivering care while remaining socially well-adjusted. It would be interesting to engage in a cost-benefit analysis of accurate empathy, and to identify the factors that regulate the respective outcomes for the person in pain and the observer of that individual.

To provide effective care, an observer must have the ability to regulate his or her own arousal and aversive self-oriented emotions (e.g., distress), because self-oriented emotions may lead observers to focus primarily upon their own needs (see Eisenberg, 2002). Effective regulation of self-oriented emotions, such as keeping distress at a moderate level, should facilitate other-oriented affective responses. Sympathy and concern for the well-being of the other person may make observers more sensitive to the consequences of their behavior, promoting flexibility in selecting and enacting particular helping behaviors attuned to the needs of the observed person in pain (Goubert et al., 2008). Health care professionals face the challenge of finding the balance that allows them to pay attention to the details of a patient's pain experience and resonate with the patient's experience without becoming emotionally overinvolved in a way that might preclude effective medical management and even lead to burnout (Larson & Yao, 2005).

A Model of the Adult Capacity for Pain-Related Empathy

The adult capacity for empathy to pain in others is the result of complex interactions between biological maturation and the individual's history of exposure to (social) events. The automatic, innate, hardwired empathic reactions to pain in others observed early in infancy become modulated by higher cognitive functions (through learning mechanisms) to ultimately reflect goal-oriented, purposeful behavior in older children and adults. The reflexive reactions to others in pain remain available, as is evident in "gut level" reactions to others who experience unexpected, sudden injury. These reactions rely primarily on the limbic system that is involved in emotional processing (Jackson, Rainville, & Decety, 2006). These are likely to be accompanied by automatic, overlearned reactions in people who are highly experienced in attending to others needing care, for example, nurses in acute care settings. Deliberative empathic responses, implying higher cognitive functions, are more likely to succeed the automatic reactions or to come into play as a response to more controlled pain displays. In particular, the verbal communication of pain, involving highly differentiated accounts of subjective experiences, may generate in listeners a complex cognitive and deep emotional appreciation of the subtleties of the sufferer's experiences. However, because verbal expression is subject to purposeful control, judgments about the credibility of the other's pain become more likely than in the case where one directly observes the other person's nonverbal pain behavior (Craig, 2007). These interactions between the type of pain reaction displayed by the person in pain and the likelihood of automatic or controlled empathic reactions by observers are illustrated in table 12.1 (Craig et al., in press).

In acute pain situations, a person's immediate pain expression is mostly automatic—including screaming, crying, facial display of pain, or escape (Hadjistavropoulos & Craig, 2002). These reactions likely elicit automatic empathic responses in observers, which have been demonstrated through the use of neuroimaging of central brain states (e.g., Lamm, Batson, & Decety, 2007; Singer et al., 2004; Simon et al., 2006). When pain persists, the

Table 12.1
Theoretical interactions between categories of pain expression (automatic/reflexive versus deliberate/intentional) and the empathic reactions of observers (uncontrolled/automatic or deliberative/reflective)

		Person in pain's expression	
		Automatic reactions (e.g., reflexive escape, facial grimaces, cry)	**Deliberate behavior** (e.g., self-report, purposive actions)
Observer's reactions	**Automatic reactions** (e.g., involuntary, viscerally experienced, motor preparation)	The uncontrolled response to acute pain is more likely to instigate involuntary empathic responses	Less likely to activate spontaneous empathy
	Deliberate behavior (e.g., contemplation or active decision making)	Reflective or contemplative consideration follows temporally	Likely to instigate reflection, questions about credibility

Note: In the Goubert et al. (2005) model of pain empathy, salient among "bottom-up" instigators is the suffering person's pain expression; whereas "top-down" determinants include the observer's (not necessarily conscious) higher-level processing of events.

situation becomes more complex, entailing more controlled processes in its communication (e.g., verbalizations of pain); some people do not want to talk about pain because they want to be seen as strong or because they fear negative social consequences (see Morley, Doyle, & Beese, 2000; Herbette & Rimé, 2004). In these circumstances, observers must exercise discretion and judgment based on a range of information that may be available.

Our model of empathy for pain groups determinants of the observer's cognitive, affective, and behavioral responses to perceiving another's pain into *bottom-up*, *top-down*, and *contextual* or *relational* factors (Goubert et al., 2005). An observer's empathic responses to another's pain are assumed to be determined by (1) characteristics of the person in pain and the availability of the cues that signal pain (these are the bottom-up determinants, such as the specifics of the pain behavior observed), (2) characteristics of the observer (these top-down determinants include higher-level decision making that reflects personal learning experiences), (3) contextual characteristics (e.g., the presence of blood, wounds, or danger in the setting), and (4) the nature of the relationship between observer and observed (e.g., professional, family, stranger). These determinants may interact in determining the observers' empathic responses.

Factors Related to the Person Observed to Be in Pain

Features of an individual's immediate reaction to physical insult, including evidence of pain and its severity (the bottom-up characteristics of the observed person), are likely to instigate empathic reactions in others. One can imagine the complex cues one might have access to when witnessing another undergoing injurious trauma: the event, such as an accident or a vicious assault; the wounds or injuries that follow; the behavioral efforts of the injured to escape or to self-protect; and the communicative behaviors that display pain for others (e.g., cries and other nonverbal vocalizations, the language of pain and distress, facial pain displays). When observers infer other people's internal experiences, they inductively use the other's behavior and affective displays to draw their inferences. However, the success rate of this bottom-up route may vary depending on the expressiveness or informativeness of the modality that conveys the bottom-up cues.

How does the broad range of cues that signify pain in others instigate empathy for others? We believe that the more spontaneous, automatic cues will have the most dramatic impact. By contrast, self-reports of pain, because they derive from personal reflection and often take the form of retrospective accounts, should typically have less impact. Of course, a good story or written account can sometimes move readers to tears, but nonverbal expressions of pain appear to be particularly potent. Recent neuroimaging studies of reactions to facial expressions of pain (e.g., Botvinick et al., 2005; Simon et al., 2006) are important because they suggest that a unique neurophysiology underlies pain empathy (Jackson, Rainville, & Decety, 2006). Among the many nonverbal cues we have mentioned, facial expression appears to provide the most specific information (Craig et al., 2001). It is noteworthy that neurophysiological reactions display substantially more powerful emotional components than sensory components in the vicarious experience of pain (Singer et al., 2004).

Individual differences in pain displays should clearly have an impact on the observer's empathic reaction. Although some people react vigorously, displaying considerable pain behavior, others rather react phlegmatically to comparable painful events. The former type may catastrophize about their personal plight (i.e., overfocus on or exaggerate the negative aspects; Sullivan et al., 2006a; Vervoort et al., 2008), whereas others may fail to perceive insidious disease or injury, misinterpret sensations as innocuous, or fail to appreciate either the costs of not seeking care or the benefits of seeking care. Sometimes, people deliberately withhold information, thereby limiting the potential for onlookers to display accurate empathy. Children ingenuously admit to suppressing pain in the interest of avoiding embarrassment in front of peers, not worrying their parents, or avoiding denial of access to play activities (Larochette, Chambers, & Craig, 2006). Complex display rules constrain and regulate the expression of pain (Zeman & Garber, 1996). People with developmental disabilities may fail to learn the skills necessary to effectively access care from others (Oberlander & Symons, 2006; Craig, 2006). Morley, Doyle, and Beese (2000) have noted the importance of disclosure or nondisclosure by persons in pain, and have observed that chronic pain patients are often unwilling to disclose. The often-reported underestimation of pain in others (Chambers et al., 1998) may reflect an active suppression of pain reporting or pain-revealing behavior, making it more difficult for observers to infer the pain. People can also be motivated to fake or exaggerate pain in the interest of personal gain (Craig & Hill, 2003), thereby creating the considerable challenge for observers of discriminating between genuine and dissembled pain displays (Hill & Craig, 2004).

Factors Related to the Observer

Our model of empathy for pain in others postulates that top-down characteristics—those pertaining to the observer—can profoundly modulate the bottom-up effects, and may be important determinants of reactions to pain in others even in the absence of any bottom-up features (see Goubert et al., 2005). First, prior experiences with particular pain situations lead to more elaborate representations of those situations in observers (see Preston & de Waal, 2002), so that empathic responses are readily elicited when another person is perceived to be in a similar situation. This influence is confirmed by the finding that patients with congenital insensitivity to pain, who are largely deprived of common stimulus-induced pain experiences, greatly underestimated the pain they observed in video clips of pain-inducing events in comparison with control subjects, especially when emotional cues were lacking (Danziger, Prkachin, & Willer, 2006). However, the results also showed that the same patients' ratings of verbally presented imaginary painful situations did not differ from those of control subjects, suggesting that a normal personal experience of pain is not necessarily required for perceiving and feeling empathy for others' pain.

Observers' ability to detect and discriminate available bottom-up information would also be expected to influence their situational empathy. For example, self-awareness with regard to one's own emotions should enhance sensitivity because the individual's recognition of his or her own feelings is the basis for identification with the feelings of others (Decety & Jackson, 2004). A recent study showed that people who scored high in alexithymia, characterized by difficulties in identifying and expressing one's own emotional states, had lower scores in their ratings of pain seen in pictures and also scored lower on questionnaires assessing their empathic capabilities (in particular, cognitive perspective taking and the capacity for other-oriented emotional responses). They also displayed poorer emotion-regulation abilities as well as decreased neural activity in brain areas involved in cognitive empathy for others' pain (Moriguchi et al., 2007).

The appraisal processes used by the observer also influence emotional responses to observing another person's pain (Lamm, Batson, & Decety, 2007). In threatening situations, such as end-stage cancer, family caregivers overestimate patient pain (Redinbaugh et al., 2002). Catastrophizing about one's own pain has been found to be related to inferences of higher pain in others (Sullivan et al., 2006b). Higher levels of emotional distress have been found in individuals who catastrophize about the pain of their spouse (Leonard & Cano, 2006) or their child (Goubert et al., 2006; Goubert et al., 2008).

Finally, while it is often assumed that gender plays a prominent role in empathy—women are believed by many to be more attentive to (Hermann, 2007) or better than men at "reading" other people's thoughts and feelings—the evidence indicates that male and female observers are equally capable of empathy, but only when both groups are sufficiently motivated (Ickes, Gesn, & Graham, 2000; Hodges & Klein, 2001).

Relational Factors

The relationship between the person in pain and the observer has been recognized as an important determinant of the observer's reactions to the other's observed or inferred distress (Craig, Lilley, & Gilbert, 1996; Vervoort et al., 2008). Closer relationships (e.g., parent-child or other family relationships) are expected to more readily elicit empathic responses (and to elicit stronger responses) than stranger or adversarial relationships. Pillai Riddell and Craig (2007) found that people who were identified as parents—but not the parents of the particular infants being described—attributed more pain in response to needle injections than did pediatricians. Nurses' responses were intermediate to, but not significantly different from, those of the parents and the pediatricians. Athough it was identified that some of the health professionals were also parents, it was argued that the lower pain estimation of (parent) professional caregivers may be due to the repetitive exposure to infants in pain, in contrast to the group of parents in this study of whom none were health professionals.

The extent to which the observing person feels a greater sense of identification with, or perceived similarity to, the suffering person might provoke a greater sense of personal "mirroring." In the social modeling literature, it is well demonstrated that similarity enhances modeling effects (Bandura, 1986). Evolutionary biologists have postulated an "affinity continuum" in terms of the degree of common genetic inheritance (Dawkins, 1976). In this view one's relatives are expected to elicit the strongest empathic reaction, which should vary in relation to the degree of kinship. At one extreme of empathic reactions would be those to dependent kin (such as one's children or parents, depending on the situation). Moving away from this extreme, the affinity continuum is posited to extend through more distant family to members of a community bound by commitment to altruistic concern and action. All these categories represent persons with whom one can identify as if they were an extension of the self, as opposed to a category of others that would include strangers, uninterested parties, competitors, antagonists, and enemies. Because in most cases family members share an intense bond and a mutual history, and because they have strong feelings of familiarity with each other, we might intuitively assume that they "know" each other and are thus able to make elaborate and individualized mental-state inferences that contribute to empathy.

Is this really the case, however? Are family members, in effect, more accurate at "reading" each other's thoughts and feelings than strangers are? Previous research by Ickes and colleagues (e.g., Simpson, Oriña, & Ickes, 2003) examined the effect of observer-target relationships on accuracy in inferring the thoughts and feelings of targets and found moderate effects. Moreover, we recently found evidence in a nonpain context that family members do not rely on relational knowledge or "inside" information about the target person to accurately infer his or her thoughts and feelings (De Corte et al., 2007). Family members were, accordingly, not more accurate than strangers were. Knowledge about the possible moderating effect of the nature or quality of the relationship between observer and observed is fragmented and scarce. This is an area that requires further investigation.

Conclusions

Empathy for pain in others has the adaptive benefit of providing information about potentially dangerous events and facilitating compassion among people in communities. The frequent reports of underestimations of other people's pain in the research literature indicate that one's ability to "know" the pain of others is far from perfect. Fully knowing the pain experience of another person—in the sense that all thoughts, feelings and sensations of the suffering person are comprehended and felt—appears impossible, for logistical and pragmatic reasons. The multiple facets of pain dictate that observers will simplify, integrate, and summarize their observations. However, cues concerning the nature of the other person's pain-related distress are often ambiguous, and observers often fail to attend to the useful information that is available (Prkachin & Craig, 1995). Further, because fully mirroring the painful distress of others could have a debilitating cognitive and emotional impact upon observers, we have argued that observers who display a moderate amount of accuracy—those who have a *sense* of knowing the experience of the other person in pain, might be the most effective caregivers.

Identifying the crucial determinants of inferences about pain in others, and the processes by which those inferences are made, is a very important task in light of its implication for the diagnosis and management of major health issues. Future investigations should take into account relational factors in order to shed light on how different relationships between observer and observed (e.g., health care provider versus parent; peer versus romantic partner) affect the perception of pain and the capacity for empathic responses.

References

Bandura, A. (1986). *Social foundations of thought and action: A social cognitive theory.* Englewood Cliffs, NJ: Prentice Hall.

Batson, C. D. (1991). *The altruism question: Toward a social-psychological answer.* Hillsdale, NJ: Erlbaum.

Botvinick, M., Jha, A. P., Bylsma, L. M., Fabian, S. A., Solomon, P. E., & Prkachin, K. M. (2005). Viewing facial expressions of pain engages cortical areas involved in the direct experience of pain. *NeuroImage, 25,* 312–319.

Chambers, C. T., Reid, G. J., Craig, K. D., McGrath, P. J., & Finley, G. A. (1998). Agreement between child and parent reports of pain. *Clinical Journal of Pain, 14,* 336–342.

Charbonneau, D., & Nicol, A. A. M. (2002). Emotional intelligence and prosocial behaviors in adolescents. *Psychological Reports, 90,* 361–370.

Craig, K. D. (2006). The construct and definition of pain in developmental disability. In F. J. Symons & T. F. Oberlander (Eds.), *Pain in individuals with developmental disabilities* (pp. 7–18). Baltimore: Paul H. Brookes.

Craig, K. D. (2007). Assessment of credibility. In R. F. Schmidt & W. D. Willis (Eds.), *Encyclopedia of pain* (pp. 491–493). New York: Springer-Verlag.

Craig, K. D., & Hill, M. L. (2003). Detecting voluntary misrepresentation of pain in facial expression. In P. Halligan, C. Bass, & D. Oakley (Eds.), *Malingering and illness deception* (pp. 336–347). Oxford: Oxford University Press.

Craig, K. D, Lilley, C. M., & Gilbert, C. A. (1996). Social barriers to optimal pain management in infants and children. *Clinical Journal of Pain, 12,* 232–242.

Craig, K. D., Prkachin, K. M., & Grunau, R. V. E. (2001). The facial expression of pain. In D. C. Turk & R. Melzack (Eds.), *Handbook of pain assessment,* 2nd ed. (pp. 153–169). New York: Guiford.

Craig, K. D.,Versloot, J., Goubert, L., Vervoort, T., & Crombez, G. (in press). Perceiving pain in others: Automatic and controlled mechanisms. *Journal of Pain.*

Danziger, N., Prkachin, K. M., & Willer, J. (2006). Is pain the price of empathy? The perception of others' pain in patients with congenital sensitivity to pain. *Brain, 129,* 2494–2507.

Davis, M. H. (1996). *Empathy: A social psychological approach.* Madison, WI: Westview Press.

Dawkins, R. (1976). *The selfish gene.* Oxford: Oxford University Press.

Decety, J., & Jackson, P. L. (2004). The functional architecture of human empathy. *Behavioral and Cognitive Neuroscience Reviews, 3,* 71–100.

De Corte, K., Buysse, A., Verhofstadt, L. L., & Devoldre, I. (2007). Empathic accuracy in families: Can family members empathize better with their intimates than strangers can? Unpublished manuscript.

Eisenberg, N. (2002). Distinctions among various modes of empathy-related reactions: A matter of importance in humans. *Behavior and Brain Sciences, 25*, 33–34.

Fiske, S. T. (1993). Controlling other people: The impact of power on stereotyping. *American Psychologist, 48*, 621–628.

Gallese, V., Keysers, C., & Rizzolatti, G. (2004). A unifying view of the basis of social cognition. *Trends in Cognitive Sciences, 8*, 396–403.

Goubert, L., Craig, K. D., Vervoort, T., Morley, S., Sullivan, M. J. L., Williams, A. C. deC., Cano, A., & Crombez, G. (2005). Facing others in pain: The effects of empathy. *Pain, 118*, 285–288.

Goubert, L., Eccleston, C., Vervoort, T., Jordan, A., & Crombez, G. (2006). Parental catastrophizing about their child's pain: The parent version of the Pain Catastrophizing Scale (PCS-P); A preliminary validation. *Pain, 123*, 254–263.

Goubert, L., Vervoort, T., Sullivan, M. J. L., Verhoeven, K., & Crombez, G. (2008). Parental emotional responses to their child's pain: the role of dispositional empathy and parental catastrophizing about their child's pain. *Journal of Pain, 9*, 272–279.

Goubert, L., Vervoort, T., & Crombez, G. (2009). Pain demands attention of others: The approach/avoidance paradox [editorial]. *Pain, 143*, 5–6.

Hadjistavropoulos, T., & Craig, K. D. (2002). A theoretical framework for understanding self-report and observational measures of pain: A communications model. *Behaviour Research and Therapy, 40*, 551–570.

Herbette, G., & Rimé, B. (2004). Verbalization of emotion in chronic pain patients and their psychological adjustment. *Journal of Health Psychology, 9*, 661–676.

Hermann, C. (2007). Modeling, social learning and pain. In R. F. Schmidt & W. D. Willis (Eds.), *The encyclopedic reference of pain* (p. 13). Heidelberg, Germany: Springer.

Hill, M. L., & Craig, K. D. (2004). Detecting deception in facial expressions of pain: Accuracy and training. *Clinical Journal of Pain, 20*, 415–422.

Hodges, S. D., & Klein, K. J. K. (2001). Regulating the costs of empathy: The price of being human. *Journal of Socio-Economics, 30*, 437–452.

Ickes, W. (2001). Measuring empathic accuracy. In J. A. Hall & F. J. Bernieri (Eds.), *Interpersonal sensitivity: Theory and measurement* (pp. 219–241). Mahwah, NJ: Erlbaum.

Ickes, W. (2003). *Everyday mind reading: Understanding what other people think and feel.* New York: Prometheus Books.

Ickes, W., Gesn, P. R., & Graham, T. (2000). Gender differences in empathic accuracy: Differential ability or differential motivation? *Personal Relationships, 7*, 95–110.

Jackson, P. L., Brunet, E., Meltzoff, A. N., & Decety, J. (2006). Empathy examined through the neural mechanisms involved in imagining how I feel versus how you feel in pain. *Neuropsychologia, 44,* 752–761.

Jackson, P. L., Rainville, P., & Decety, J. (2006). To what extent do we share the pain of others? Insight from the neural bases of pain empathy. *Pain, 125,* 5–9.

Jussim, L. (1991). Social perception and social reality: A reflector-construction model. *Psychological Review, 98,* 54–73.

Lamm, C., Batson, C. D., & Decety, J. (2007). The neural substrate of human empathy: Effects of perspective-taking and cognitive appraisal. *Journal of Cognitive Neuroscience, 19,* 42–58.

Langford, D. J., Crager, S. E., Shehzad, Z., Smith, S. B., Sotocinal, S. G., Levenstadt, J. S., Chanda, M. L., Levitin, D. J., & Mogil, J. S. (2006). Social modulation of pain as evidence for empathy in mice. *Science, 312,* 1967–1970.

Larochette, A. C., Chambers, C. T., & Craig, K. D. (2006). Genuine, suppressed and faked facial expressions of pain in children. *Pain, 126,* 64–71.

Larson, E. B., & Yao, C. (2005). Clinical empathy as emotional labor in the patient-physician relationship. *Journal of the American Medical Association, 293,* 1100–1106.

Leonard, M. T., & Cano A. (2006). Pain affects spouses too: Personal experience with pain and catastrophizing as correlates of spouse distress. *Pain, 126,* 139–146.

Levenson, R. W., & Ruef, A. M. (1992). Empathy: A physiological substrate. *Journal of Personality and Social Psychology, 63,* 234–246.

Moriguchi, Y., Decety, J., Ohnishi, T., Maeda, M., Mori, T., Nemoto, K., Matsuda, H., & Komaki, G. (2007). Empathy and judging others' pain: An fMRI study of alexithymia. *Cerebral Cortex, 17,* 2223–2234.

Morley, S., Doyle, K., & Beese, A. (2000). Talking to others about pain: Suffering in silence. In M. Devor, M. C. Rowbotham, & Z. Wiesenfeld-Hallin (Eds.), *Proceedings of the Ninth World Congress on Pain* (vol. 16, pp. 1123–1129). Seattle, WA: International Association for the Study of Pain.

Merskey, H., & Bogduk, N. (1994). Part III: Pain Terms, A current list with definitions and notes on usage. In H. Merskey, & N. Bogduk (Eds.), *Classification of chronic pain, second edition, IASP Task Force on Taxonomy* (pp. 209–214). Seattle: IASP Press.

Oberlander, T. F., & Symons, F. J. (2006). *Pain in children with developmental disabilities.* Baltimore, MD: Brookes.

Palm, K. M., Polusny, M. A., Follette, V. M. (2004). Vicarious traumatization: Potential hazards and interventions for disaster and trauma workers. *Prehospital and Disaster Medicine, 19,* 73–78.

Pillai Riddell, R. R., & Craig, K. D. (2007). Judgments of infant pain: The impact of caregiver identity and infant age. *Journal of Pediatric Psychology, 32,* 501–511.

Preston, S. D., & de Waal, F. B. M. (2002). Empathy: Its ultimate and proximate bases. *Behavioral and Brain Sciences, 25,* 1–72.

Prkachin, K. M., & Craig, K. D. (1995). Expressing pain: The communication and interpretation of facial-pain signals. *Journal of Nonverbal Behavior, 19*, 191–205.

Redinbaugh, E. M., Baum, A., DeMoss, C., Fello, M., & Arnold, R. (2002). Factors associated with the accuracy of family caregiver estimates of patient pain. *Journal of Pain and Symptom Management, 23*, 31–38.

Schaller, M., & Cialdini, R. D. (1988). The economics of empathic helping: Support for a mood management motive. *Journal of Experimental Social Psychology, 24*, 163–181.

Simon, D., Craig, K. D., Miltner, W. H. R., & Rainville, P. (2006). Brain responses to dynamic facial expressions of pain. *Pain, 126*, 309–318.

Simpson, J. A., Oriña, M. M., & Ickes, W. (2003). When accuracy hurts, and when it helps: A test of the empathic accuracy model in martial interactions. *Journal of Personality and Social Psychology, 85*, 881–893.

Singer, T., Seymour, B., O'Doherty, J., Kaube, H., Dolan, R. J., & Frith, C. D. (2004). Empathy for pain involves the affective but not sensory components of pain. *Science, 303*, 1157–1162.

Sullivan, M. J. L., Martel, M. O., Tripp, D. A., Savard, A., & Crombez, G. (2006a). The relation between catastrophizing and the communication of pain experience. *Pain, 122*, 282–288.

Sullivan, M. J. L., Martel, M. O., Tripp, D. A., Savard, A., & Crombez, G. (2006b). Catastrophic thinking and heightened perception of pain in others. *Pain, 123*, 37–44.

Vervoort, T., Craig, K. D., Goubert, L., Dehoorne, J., Joos, R., Matthys, D., Buysse, A., & Crombez, G. (2008). Expressive dimensions of pain catastrophizing: A comparative analysis of school children and children with clinical pain. *Pain, 134*, 59–68.

Williams, A. C. deC., & Craig, K. D. (2006). A science of pain expression? *Pain, 125*, 202–203.

Zeman, J., & Garber, J. (1996). Display rules for anger, sadness, and pain: It depends on who is watching. *Child Development, 67*, 957–973.

IV Evolutionary and Neuroscience Perspectives on Empathy

13 Neural and Evolutionary Perspectives on Empathy

C. Sue Carter, James Harris, and Stephen W. Porges

This chapter examines autonomic and neuroendocrine processes that have been implicated in social behaviors and emotional states, including those assumed to reflect empathy in humans. The word is derived from the Greek and literally means "to suffer with." However, as a psychological construct, empathy has been used to describe a broader range of feelings, expressions, and behaviors that enable individuals to recognize, to perceive, and to respond appropriately to the emotional state of others. Although it has been argued that empathy is a unique characteristic of human consciousness, emotional contagion (Hatfield, Rapson, & Le, this volume) and consolation have been demonstrated in other mammalian species, including social primate species, and especially bonobo chimpanzees (Preston & de Waal, 2002).

If operationally defined to include contingent social responses to emotional expressions of pain, fear, or hunger (such as isolation calls and hunger cries), then empathy is an important adaptive behavior within the repertoire of all mammals. We propose that empathy is a feature shared by humans with other mammals that is dependent on the neural circuits that emerged during the evolutionary transition from reptiles to mammals. The neural and chemical building blocks of empathy are evolutionarily conserved and shared across mammalian species, and they differ significantly from those in our reptilian ancestors.

In contemporary cognitive neuroscience, empathy is most often represented as a function of higher brain structures, including the cortex (Decety & Jackson, 2004; Lamm, Batson, & Decety, 2007). However, at least some of the underlying physiological substrates necessary for the expression of empathy are shared with more general aspects of emotionality, as well as sociability and reproduction, which are dependent on lower brain structures and the autonomic nervous system. An understanding of feelings and emotions requires an awareness of the neural and endocrine systems necessary for both detection of and response to bodily states (Porges, 1997, 2007). Thus, empathy also can be viewed in terms of adaptive neuroendocrine and autonomic processes, including changes in neuromodulatory systems that regulate bodily states, emotions, and reactivity.

Social behaviors are best understood in the context of evolution. Both mutual aid among members of a species and survival of the fittest arose as products of evolution. The genetically fittest or reproductively most successful individuals also may be those who engage in mutual aid or social support (Kropotkin, 1989). This position was taken by early Russian evolutionists, who proposed that greater emphasis should be placed on mutual aid or cooperation, rather than simply on individual survival (Todes, 1989; Harris, 2003).

During most of the twentieth century, there was resistance to considering social behavior and benefits to others, especially nonrelatives, as a major factor in evolution. However, recently there has been increasing support for the notion that selection could act at the level of the group as well as at the individual level (Wilson & Sober, 1989; MacLean, 1990). Thus, social behavior and the benefits of sociality are now understood as central to evolution (Nowak, 2006; Harris, 2007). Species-typical patterns of sociality and their mechanisms are products of evolution. Analysis of the phylogenetic origins of human social behavior provides a critical perspective for understanding empathy.

An Evolving Autonomic and Social Nervous System

The evolutionary state of the nervous system, especially the brain, the autonomic nervous system, and the bidirectional neural pathways that communicate between the brain and the autonomic nervous system, influences the range of emotional expression and affect awareness that is possible in humans; this spectrum of capability in turn determines the quality of social communication (Porges, 2007). The biology of social behavior also is supported by and interwoven with autonomic, endocrine, and other homeostatic processes responsible for survival. Basic to survival is the capacity to react to challenges or stressors and maintain visceral homeostatic states necessary for vital processes such as oxygenation of tissues and supply of nutrients to the body. For these reasons, the neural circuits involved in regulating social interactions overlap with those that regulate visceral homeostasis to support health.

The autonomic nervous system is fundamental to affective experience, emotional expression, facial gestures, vocal communication, and contingent social behavior. Refined neural pathways have developed to support the needs of mammalian communication and selective sociality. (Figure 13.1 represents this system schematically.)

Consistent with these phylogenetic changes were changes in the neural regulation of the autonomic nervous system, delineated in table 13.1.

Specifically, as mammals emerged from their reptilian ancestors, the autonomic nervous system changed to support increased metabolic demands. With the evolution of mammals, a new ventral vagal efferent pathway emerged to play a major role in cardiac regulation. This comparatively modern vagal pathway provided a neuroanatomical and neurophysiological link between the brain stem regulation of the striated muscles of the face and the regulation of the autonomic nervous system.

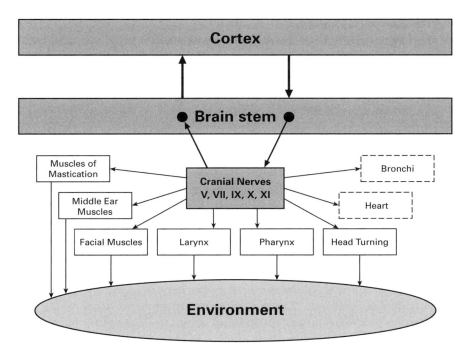

Figure 13.1

The social engagement system. Social communication is determined by the cortical regulation of medullary nuclei via corticobulbar pathways. The social engagement system consists of a somatomotor component (i.e., special visceral efferent pathways that regulate the striated muscles of the face and head) and a visceromotor component (i.e., the myelinated vagus that regulates the heart and bronchi). Solid rectangles indicate the somatomotor component. Dashed rectangles indicate the visceromotor component.

Table 13.1

Phylogenetic states of the polyvagal theory

Stage	ANS component	Behavioral function
III	Myelinated vagus (ventral vagal complex)	Social communication, self-soothing and calming, inhibition of sympathetic-adrenal influences
II	Sympathetic-adrenal system (sympathetic nervous system)	Mobilization (fight/flight, active avoidance)
I	Unmyelinated vagus (dorsal vagal complex)	Immobilization (death feigning, passive avoidance, behavioral shutdown)

The Evolution of the Human Head and Face

During the transition from primitive synapsids (mammal-like reptiles) to living mammals, neural and anatomical structures necessary for social communication were made possible by evolutionary modifications in cranial anatomy. Central to these systems were cranial nerves with origins in the brain stem. The autonomic nervous system, as well as the physical elements of the human face including the nerves and muscles necessary for facial gestures and auditory communication, evolved from primitive gill arches. Complex social behaviors became possible through the emergence of the mammalian autonomic nervous system which also supported the oxygenation of blood, allowing the development of a larger mammalian cortex.

Mammals are highly dependent on audition for social communication. Unique to the mammalian auditory system is the specialized mammalian middle ear, which evolved from primitive vertebrate gill arches. As the cortex expanded, requiring a larger and more flexible cranium, three small middle-ear bones detached from the mandibular arch. These tiny bones, modified to form the mammalian middle ear, together amplify and internally direct low-amplitude sound waves. The middle ear permits detection of high-frequency airborne sounds (i.e., sounds in the frequency of human voice), even when the acoustic environment is dominated by low-frequency sounds. The development of the mammalian middle ear also was critical in the evolutionary history of sociality because it allowed the mother to eat, nurse, and listen to conspecific vocalizations at the same time.

Concurrent with these evolutionary modifications, muscles and peripheral nerves of the face and head took on functions that allowed control over speech and listening (figure 13.1). A link evolved between the neural regulation of the muscles of the face and head and a new myelinated vagus (with faster transmission than its unmyelinated counterpart). This more modern component of the vagus efficiently fostered calm behavioral states and dampened the reactivity of the sympathetic nervous system and the hypothalamic-pituitary-adrenal (HPA) axis (Porges, 2007). Thus, sociality could overcome states of fear.

Connecting the Head and the Heart

The mammalian nervous system evolved with an ability to signal and to detect vocalizations reflecting states such as pain, distress, or joy. The neural regulation of larynx and pharynx was consistent with the functions of the middle ear and allowed a "vagal brake" that could regulate visceral state. Thus, a coordinated system exists with a clearly defined and functional "face-heart" connection (Porges, 2003). In mammals this system allowed a total body response to external cues, especially those broadcast through an auditory modality. As a result of these adaptations, mammals have a unique capacity to respond contingently to the acoustic features of pain and joy. Although the critical role of auditory communication in mammalian behavior is well established, less is known about the role of auditory cues in emotion, in part because most laboratory studies of emotion have focused on evaluating the aversive nature of visual stimuli in empathic behavior.

Empathy and the Evolution of Social Awareness in Mammals

Empathy is defined by reactions to others, usually of our own species. As a hypothetical construct, it assumes the capacity to distinguish between inanimate objects and conspecifics. This distinction, between reacting to an object and reacting to conspecifics, provides the neural basis for a discussion of empathy within the context of a mammalian social nervous system. The phylogenetic emergence of a mammalian social nervous system, characterized by a "face-heart" connection, sets the neurophysiological platform for social communication that requires not only contingent behaviors, but also mental and visceral role-playing. The concept of empathy accounts for the phylogenetic advantages of these systems in promoting cooperative behaviors that enable *groups* of individuals to share in the responsibility for detecting danger and to facilitate social communication and social interactions within a *safe* environment. It is this ability to share knowledge regarding environmental danger that provides the basis for the subsequent development of social groups, societies, and their products. Thus, in articulating the neurobiology of empathy we are led directly to the neural circuits that have enabled individuals to detect and respond to the features that identify another person as both living and safe.

Because empathy is linked to feelings contingent on the detection of distress in others, the concept of empathy can be further understood by examining neural mechanisms that mediate both the expression of feelings and the detection of feelings in others. Uniquely mammalian neural circuits exist to allow facial expression and vocal intonation. In addition, the capacity to detect and respond to these features in others relies on specialized neural circuits, permitting rapid, contingent responses to the feelings of others (Adolphs, 2006).

Critical to understanding the concept of empathy is an awareness of the capacity of the nervous system to detect and evaluate the features of the social environment. At the heart of mammalian survival is the concept of safety and the ability to distinguish whether the environment is safe, and whether other individuals are friend or foe.

The same neural systems that regulate survival and homeostasis are associated with specific neurobehavioral states that limit the extent to which a mammal can be physically approached and whether it can communicate or establish new relationships. To accurately evaluate another individual, it is necessary to assess the characteristics of the other. If the result is positive, then the mammalian nervous system must inhibit defensive responses in deference to social engagement strategies. But how does the nervous system know when the environment is safe, dangerous, or life threatening, and what neural mechanisms evaluate risk in the environment?

The neural evaluation of risk is rapid and can occur without conscious awareness. For that reason the term *neuroception* has been introduced to describe how neural circuits that function as a safety-threat detection system are capable of distinguishing among situations that are safe, dangerous, or life threatening (table 13.1) (Porges, 2003).

Under conditions of perceived safety, primitive limbic structures that control fight, flight, or freeze behaviors are inhibited, using mechanisms that are dependent upon subcortical limbic structures. New neural systems evolved in mammals that involved cortical regulation of subcortical structures and, in many instances, co-opted the defense functions of primitive structures to support other functions including those related to reproductive behavior and selective social interactions (Porges, 1998). As discussed in the next section, hormones may allow neural systems that were previously involved in defensive functions to be co-opted for prosocial actions.

Functionally, when the environment is perceived as safe, two important features are expressed. First, the bodily state is regulated in an efficient manner to promote growth, restoration, and visceral homeostasis. This is done through an increase in the influence of myelinated, more evolutionarily modern and rapid, vagal motor pathways on the cardiac pacemaker. When activated this mechanism slows the heart, inhibits the fight/flight mechanisms of the sympathetic nervous system, and dampens the stress response system of the HPA-axis (e.g., cortisol); this system even reduces inflammation by modulating immune reactions (e.g., cytokines). Second, through the process of evolution, the brain stem nuclei that regulate the myelinated vagus became integrated with the nuclei that regulate the muscles of the face and head. This link resulted in bidirectional coupling between spontaneous social engagement behaviors and bodily states. Specifically, the visceral states that promote growth and restoration are linked neuroanatomically and neurophysiologically with the muscles that regulate components of eye gaze, facial expression, listening, and prosody (figure 13.1) (Porges, 2001; 2007).

Functional neuroimaging methods have identified specific neural structures that are involved in detecting risk. These studies suggest that two areas of the temporal cortex, the fusiform gyrus and the superior temporal sulcus, are involved in evaluating biological movement and intention—including the detection of features such as movements, vocalizations, and faces—that contribute to an individual being perceived as safe or trustworthy (Adolphs, 2006). Slight changes in these stimuli can either pose threat or signal safety. Connectivity between these areas of the temporal cortex and the amygdala suggests a top-down control in the processing of facial features that could actively inhibit activity of the structures involved in the expression of defensive strategies.

The human nervous system, like those of other mammals, did not evolve solely to survive in safe environments, but also to cope with danger and promote survival in life-threatening contexts. To accomplish this adaptive flexibility, the human nervous system retained two more primitive neural circuits to regulate defensive strategies (i.e., the fight/flight and freeze behaviors). It is important to note that social behavior, social communication, and visceral homeostasis are largely incompatible with the neurophysiological states and behaviors that are activated by the two neural circuits that support defense strategies.

Three neural circuits have evolved in a phylogenetically organized hierarchy. The newest circuit, which includes features of empathy, is used first. When that circuit fails to provide safety we recruit the older defensive circuits, including fight/flight and then freezing/immo-bilization, sequentially. As mammals evolved they became dependent on social cues and social support from others, usually of their own species. Social behaviors facilitate both survival and reproduction, allowing mammals to more safely eat, digest, sleep, mate, and care for their dependent young. These same factors, which led to the evolution of mammalian social communication, were involved in the evolution of the primate autonomic nervous system and presumably play a role in the capacity to experience emotions, including empathic feelings, and to exhibit empathic responses.

Neuroendocrine Correlates of Sociality

Young mammals are dependent on their mothers for nourishment. The resulting interaction between the mother and infant may be a physiological and neuroendocrine prototype for mammalian sociality. The circuits involved offer the potential for selective responding to specific other members of the species, such as a mother to her offspring, that did not exist in the reptilian ancestors of modern mammals.

Mammalian neuropeptide hormones, including oxytocin and vasopressin, act throughout the brain and body to integrate many processes including social behaviors, emotional feelings and responses, and the autonomic nervous system. Oxytocin is of particular importance to mammals because it facilitates mammalian birth, lactation, and the development of maternal behaviors and social bonds. We hypothesize here that these neuroendocrine processes, acting at various sites in the nervous system already implicated more generally in sociality and social communication, also underlie the behavioral states and responses necessary for empathy.

In this context, it is not surprising that social interactions and isolation have powerful physiological consequences. The need for social interactions has been documented by a growing body of evidence suggesting that individuals with a perceived sense of social support are more likely to avoid or survive illness and have longer lives than otherwise similar people who live alone or who experience a sense of loneliness (Cacioppo et al., 2006). It seems likely that the processes that change during isolation are related to those involved in empathy.

Empathy as identified in humans may or may not exist in nonprimates, particularly rodents, the most common models for neurobiological research. However, the underlying substrates for sociality or sociability (versus defensive reactions), are shared among mammalian species. Although neuroendocrine processes that are specific to empathy remain to be described, it is likely that various forms of mammalian sociality share common substrates. For example, adult social bonds are based on at least some of the same processes that are necessary for maternal behavior, selective maternal bonds, and the management of stressful experiences (Carter & Keverne, 2002).

Fundamental to social behaviors, including parental behaviors, sociality between adults, and empathy, are the processes that regulate approach or avoidance toward another individual. At the most basic level, sensory, autonomic, emotional, and motor systems are primed to allow the organism to approach or withdraw. Sensory and emotional processes are tuned to detect and interpret the features of social cues and to respond with autonomic reactions and appropriate motor patterns. And selective social and emotional responses, including those necessary for social relationships, usually are implicit in the expression of empathy.

Highly Social Mammals and the Analysis of Prosocial Behaviors

One approach to understanding the neurobiology of positive social behaviors has been to examine interspecies differences in sociality among mammals. Socially monogamous species share with humans a set of physiological and behavioral characteristics including the capacity to form social bonds and develop extended families, usually consisting of a male and female pair and their offspring (Carter, DeVries, & Getz, 1995). Socially monogamous rodents, such as prairie voles, are especially sensitive to their social environment and may offer a particularly powerful model for understanding the mechanisms that enable positive social experiences.

Neuropeptides and Selective Sociality

Studies of social bond formation in prairie voles have been helpful for understanding the behavioral, neuroendocrine and autonomic effects of two neuropeptide hormones—oxytocin and vasopressin—that are important to mammalian sociality. Oxytocin probably played a pivotal role in the evolution of primates. As the central nervous systems and skulls of primates expanded, mechanisms evolved to facilitate birth and postnatal nourishment for the infant (Carter & Altemus, 1997). Oxytocin facilitates the birth process through powerful muscle contraction. It may even protect the fetal nervous system during the birth (Tyzio et al., 2006). Oxytocin also facilitates milk ejection and thus lactation. Lactation in turn permits the birth of immature infants, allowing postnatal cortical and intellectual development in young that are dependent on their mother as a source of both food and caregiving.

Oxytocin also sits at the center of a neuroendocrine network that coordinates social behaviors and concurrent response to various stressors, generally acting to reduce reactivity to stressors (Carter, 1998). Oxytocin tends to decrease fear and anxiety and to increase tolerance for stressful stimuli. Oxytocin may protect the vulnerable mammalian nervous system from regressing into the primitive states of lower brain stem dominance (such as the "reptile-like" freezing pattern with an associated shutdown of higher neural processes); mammals—with their comparatively large cortexes and a corresponding need for high levels of oxygen—cannot endure long periods of hypoxia (Porges, 2007). At the same time oxytocin appears to encourage various forms of sociality (Carter, 2007).

Oxytocin is released and works in conjunction with a related neuropeptide known as vasopressin. Vasopressin is structurally similar to oxytocin, differing by only two of nine amino acids. The genes that regulate the synthesis of these peptides are modifications of a common ancestral gene. The similarity of the oxytocin and vasopressin molecules also allows them to influence each other's receptors. The actions of oxytocin and vasopressin are often—but not always—in opposite directions. Oxytocin tends to reduce behavioral and autonomic reactivity to stressful experiences, whereas vasopressin is associated with arousal and vigilance. Vasopressin also plays a role in social behaviors and has adaptive functions in the face of behavioral and physiological stressors (Carter, 2007).

Various brain stem neural systems, including those that rely on peptides such as oxytocin and vasopressin, help to regulate emotional states including approach-avoidance reactions and the tendency of mammals to immobilize (Porges, 1998). Oxytocin and vasopressin are synthesized in and are particularly abundant in the hypothalamus, but they may reach distant receptors including those in the cortex and in lower brain stem areas, such as the dorsal motor nucleus, responsible for autonomic functions, thus helping to integrate behavioral and emotional responses.

Oxytocin and vasopressin have the capacity to move through the brain by diffusion, rather than acting only across a synapse or requiring transport by the circulatory system; for this reason these neuropeptides have pervasive effects on the central nervous system. Oxytocin in particular is unique in having only one known receptor and in using the same receptor for many functions, thus allowing coordinated effects on behavior and physiology. Vasopressin has three subtypes of receptors. One, the V1a receptor, has been implicated in various kinds of social and defensive behaviors; it also helps to regulate blood pressure. Dynamic interactions between oxytocin and vasopressin may be of particular importance to the approach and avoidance components of sociality. Intranasal oxytocin facilitates "trust" behavior as measured in a computer game (Kosfeld et al., 2005) and the ability to detect subtle cues from pictures of eyes (Domes et al., 2007). These studies support the hypothesis that oxytocin may have a role in the behavioral responses necessary for empathy.

The importance of social interactions can be understood in part by examining the consequences of placing animals in social isolation. For example, prolonged isolation is associated with increases in oxytocin (Grippo, Gerena, et al., 2007). Elevated oxytocin in this context may be protective against the negative consequences of isolation. There is also evidence that opioids and dopamine, probably through interactions with oxytocin and vasopressin, influence social behavior and specifically social bonds (Carter and Keverne, 2002; Aragona et al., 2006). Thus, social interactions have powerful effects on reward systems, possibly contributing to the emotional effects associated with empathic responses.

Prairie voles also have a human-like autonomic nervous system, characterized by high levels of vagal efferent activity through the myelinated vagal pathways that regulate the heart (Grippo, Lamb, et al., 2007). Unlike domestic mice or rats—species with comparatively low cardiac vagal tone—the prairie vole provides a model in which the branch of the vagus involved in the "face-heart" connection is a potent regulator of autonomic state. Thus, highly social mammals like prairie voles may serve as models for understanding the role of the autonomic nervous system and visceral reactions in social behavior. Consistent with this expectation, in the prairie vole isolation produces profound reductions in vagal control of the heart, increases in sympathetic arousal, and a reduced capacity to recover after a stressor, especially in the face of social stress (Grippo, Gerena, et al., 2007). Oxytocin injections are capable of reversing the cardiac effects of isolation (Grippo, Carter, & Porges, unpublished data).

Oxytocin and vasopressin receptors are found in many limbic structures, including the extended amygdala. The amygdala and its connections serve a role in the integration of reactions to various kinds of sensory stimuli, including approach and avoidance (Davis, 2006). In human males, intranasal administration of oxytocin inhibited the activity of the amygdala and altered downstream connections to brain stem structures involved in the regulation of the autonomic nervous system (Kirsch et al., 2005). Vasopressin, acting centrally (in areas including the bed nucleus of the stria terminalis [BNST], amygdala, and lateral septum), may elevate vigilance and defensiveness, possibly serving in some cases as an antagonist to the effects of oxytocin. Behaviors mediated by the central amygdala may mediate stimulus-specific fear, while the BNST has been implicated in experiences related to anxiety. Other peptides, including corticotropin-releasing factor (CRF), released during "stressful" experiences may be anxiogenic, acting in the extended amygdala, including the BNST, to influence responses to dangerous or threatening cues (Davis, 2006). At least some of the fear-associated or defensive actions of CRF or vasopressin can be counteracted by oxytocin. Thus, oxytocin may have the capacity to reduce fear and calm the sympathetic responses to stressful stimuli.

Possible Mechanisms for Sex Differences in Sociality or Empathy

It is reported that females are more empathic than males (for a review see Chakrabarti and Baron-Cohen, 2006). Explanations for sex differences typically focus on steroid hormones. However, neuropeptides also may be involved. For example, the hypothalamic synthesis of vasopressin is androgen dependent, and this molecule may be of particular importance to behavior in males. Oxytocin is estrogen dependent but has functions in both males and females. Working together these molecules may allow sexually dimorphic responses to tasks involving contradictory affective states such as those involved in forming social bonds or showing empathy, while simultaneously expressing defensive or aggressive behaviors. In addition, oxytocin receptors have been found in midbrain regions that organize defensive motor behaviors and autonomic states and are assumed to down-regulate these circuits under conditions of safety. These and other findings predict sex differences in the substrates for empathy.

Elevations in oxytocin during periods of isolation in prairie voles are also sexually dimorphic, with females more likely than males to show increases in oxytocin (Grippo, Gerena, et al., 2007). In human females increases in oxytocin were associated with "gaps in social relationship" (Taylor et al., 2006). The significance of isolation-related elevations in oxytocin remains to be empirically determined, but it is likely that oxytocin is a component of a homeostatic process that helps mammals deal with isolation or other stressful experiences. Such responses might also facilitate preparedness for social engagement or enhance feelings of empathy, functions that might be especially adaptive in females, who may be less able than males to cope with isolation. In the context of personal safety, the release of oxytocin could encourage social interactions including those associated with detecting and responding to the emotions or experiences of others.

Vasopressin, because of its sexually dimorphic occurrence in the extended amygdala and lateral septum (levels are higher in males) is also a candidate for a role in explaining sex differences in empathy. For example, males and females might experience or respond to empathy-eliciting stimuli using sexually dimorphic neural pathways.

Summary and Predictions

Emotional and visceral states influence how we feel about and react to others, and thus our capacity for empathy. Awareness of factors that regulate emotional responses and feeling lead us to a deeper understanding of the evolved neurobiology of empathy. For example, visceral sensations make up an important component of empathy. Visceral sensations in turn represent the communication between visceral organs (e.g., heart and gut) and the brain stem, through the autonomic nervous system. The autonomic nervous system is a bidirectional system, including both sensory and motor components. Brain stem structures involved in the regulation of autonomic state are sentries of visceral states and feelings, and they also convey defensive signals, including emotional cues, to the periphery. The brain stem also provides a portal through which sensory information related to peripheral sensations, including social cues, contributes to the general activation of higher brain structures including the cortex. Thus, visceral regulation can be mediated by brain stem systems that control the heart and gut, and also can convey sensory information to the brain stem. Brain stem structures in turn transmit information to brain regions, such as the insula, that both regulate autonomic state and convey features of this activation to higher brain structures (Critchley et al., 2006).

Selective social behaviors can facilitate survival and reproduction, promoting safety and a sense of emotional security. Sociality is essential to human existence, and it is likely that the neural substrates and hormonal conditions that permit empathy are shared with those that enable other forms of sociality including willingness to approach or "trust" others (Kosfeld et al., 2005) and sensitivity to the emotions of others (Domes et al., 2007). A sense of trust and sensitivity to social cues are likely elements of empathy. Neural systems, including autonomic functions, that rely on brain stem neuropeptides, such as oxytocin and vasopressin, are plausible correlates for empathy. Oxytocin is a putative mediator of empathy, especially if the behavioral reactions involve immobilization without fear (Porges, 1998).

Alternatively, vasopressin might be implicated in situations where a more active strategy is required for an effective response. There is evidence from other situations that vasopressin has different effects in males and females (Thompson et al., 2006), and vasopressin may be of more importance in males than in females (Carter, 2007).

The strategy of investigating empathy by examining the neural systems that rely on brain stem neuropeptides could be extended to the level of genetic analysis. For example, the genetic substrates responsible for the production of oxytocin and vasopressin receptors have been linked to disorders such as autism (Jacob et al., 2007). Individual or sex differences in the genetics of these systems might be associated with individual differences in the capacity for or the experience of empathy. The connections suggested here await further experimental testing.

References

Adolphs, R. (2006). How do we know the minds of others? Domain-specificity, simulation, and enactive social cognition. *Brain Research, 1079,* 25–35.

Aragona, B. J., Liu, Y., Yu, Y. J., Curtis, J. T., Detwiler, J. M., Insel, T. R., & Wang, Z. (2006). Nucleus accumbens dopamine differentially mediates the formation and maintenance of monogamous pair bonds. *Nature Neuroscience, 9,* 133–139.

Cacioppo, J. T., Hughes, M. E., Waite, L. J., Hawkely, L. C., & Thisted, R. A. (2006). Loneliness as a specific risk factor for depressive symptoms: Cross-sectional and longitudinal analysis. *Psychology of Aging, 21,* 140–151.

Carter, C. S. (1998). Neuroendocrine perspectives on social attachment and love. *Psychoneuroendocrinology, 23,* 779–818.

Carter, C. S. (2003). Developmental consequences of oxytocin. *Physiology and Behavior, 79,* 383–397.

Carter, C. S. (2007). Sex differences in oxytocin and vasopressin: Implications for autism spectrum disorders? *Behavioural Brain Research, 176,* 170–186.

Carter, C. S., & Altemus, M. (1997). Integrative functions of lactational hormones in social behavior and stress management. *Annals of the New York Academy of Sciences, 807,* 164–174.

Carter, C. S., DeVries, A. C., & Getz, L. L. (1995). Physiological substrates of mammalian monogamy: The prairie vole model. *Neuroscience and Biobehavioral Reviews, 19,* 303–314.

Carter, C. S., & Keverne, E. B. (2002). The neurobiology of social affiliation and pair bonding. In D. Pfaff, A. Etgan, et al. (Eds.), *Hormones, Brain, and Behavior* (Vol. 1, pp. 299–335). San Diego, CA: Academic Press.

Chakrabarti, B., & Baron-Cohen, S. (2006). Empathizing: Neurocognitive developmental mechanisms and individual differences. *Progress in Brain Research, 156,* 403–417.

Critchley, H. D., Wiens, S., Rotshtein, P., Öhman, A., & Dolan, R. J. (2004). Neural systems supporting interoceptive awareness. *Nature Neuroscience, 7,* 189–195.

Davis, M. (2006). Neural systems involved in fear and anxiety measured with fear-potentiated startle. *American Psychologist, 61,* 741–756.

Decety, J., & Jackson, P. L. (2004). The functional architecture of human empathy. *Behavioral and Cognitive Neuroscience Reviews, 3,* 71–100.

Domes, G., Heinrichs, M., Michel, A., Berger, C., & Herpertz, S. C. (2007). Oxytocin improves "mind-reading" in humans. *Biological Psychiatry, 61,* 731–733.

Grippo, A. J., Gerena, D., Huang, J., Kumar, N., Shah, M., Ughreja, R., & Carter, C. S. (2007b) Social isolation induces behavioral and neuroendocrine disturbances relevant to depression in female and male prairie voles. *Psychoneuroendocrinology, 32,* 966–980.

Grippo, A. J., Lamb, D. G., Carter, C. S., & Porges, S. W. (2007a). Cardiac regulation in the socially monogamous prairie vole. *Physiology and Behavior, 90,* 386–393.

Harris, J. C. (2003). Social neuroscience, empathy, brain integration, and neurodevelopmental disorders. *Physiology and Behavior, 79,* 525–531.

Harris, J. C. (2007). The evolutionary neurobiology, emergence and facilitation of empathy. In T. F. D. Farrow & P. W. R. Woodruff, *Empathy in mental illness.* New York: Cambridge University Press.

Jacob, S., Brune, C. W., Carter, C. S., Leventhal, B. L., Lord, C., & Cook, E. H., Jr. (2007). Association of the oxytocin receptor gene (OXTR) in Caucasian children and adolescents with autism. *Neuroscience Letters, 417,* 6–9.

Kirsch, P., Esslinger, C., Chen, Q., Mier, D., Lis, S., Siddhanti, S., Gruppe, H., Mattay, V. S., Gallhofer, B., & Meyer-Lindenberg, A. (2005). Oxytocin modulates neural circuitry for social cognition and fear in humans. *Journal of Neuroscience, 25,* 11489–11493.

Kosfeld, M., Heinrichs, M., Zak, P. J., Fischbacher, U., & Fehr, E. (2005). Oxytocin increases trust in humans. *Nature, 435,* 673–676.

Kropotkin, P. I. (1989). *Mutual aid: A factor in evolution.* Montreal: Black Rose.

Lamm, C., Batson, C. D., & Decety, J. (2007). The neural substrate of human empathy: Effects of perspective-taking and cognitive appraisal. *Journal of Cognitive Neuroscience, 19,* 42–58.

MacLean, P. D. (1990). *The triune brain in evolution: Role in paleocerebral functions.* New York: Plenum Press.

Nowak, M. A. (2006). Five rules for the evolution of cooperation. *Science, 314,* 1560–1563.

Porges, S. W. (1997). Emotion: An evolutionary by-product of the neural regulation of the autonomic nervous system. *Annals of the New York Academy of Sciences, 807,* 62–77.

Porges, S. W. (1998). Love: An emergent property of the mammalian autonomic nervous system. *Psychoneuroendocrinology, 23,* 837–861.

Porges, S. W. (2001). The polyvagal theory: phylogenetic substrates of a social nervous system. *International Journal of Psychophysiology, 42,* 123–146.

Porges, S. W. (2003). Social engagement and attachment: A phylogenetic perspective. *Annals of the New York Academy of Sciences, 1008,* 31–47.

Porges, S. W. (2007). The polyvagal perspective. *Biological Psychology, 74,* 116–143.

Preston, S. D., & de Waal, F. B. (2002). Empathy: Its ultimate and proximate bases. *Behavioral and Brain Sciences, 25,* 1–20.

Taylor, S. E., Gonzaga, G. C., Klein, L.C., Hu, P., Greendale, G. A., & Seeman, T. E. (2006). Relation of oxytocin to psychological stress responses and hypothalamic-pituitary-adrenocortical axis activity in older women. *Psychosomatic Medicine, 68,* 238–245.

Thompson, R. R., George, K., Walton, J. C., Orr S. P., & Benson, J. (2006). Sex-specific influences of vasopressin on human social communication. *Proceedings of the National Academy of Sciences USA, 103,* 7889–7894.

Todes, D. P. (1989). *Darwin without Malthus: The struggle for existence in Russian evolutionary thought.* New York: Oxford University Press.

Tyzio, R., Cossart, R., Khalilov, I., Minlebaev, M., Hubner, C. A., Represa, A., Ben-Ari, Y., & Khazipov, R. (2006). Maternal oxytocin triggers a transient inhibitory switch in GABA signaling in the fetal brain during delivery. *Science, 314,* 1788–1792.

Wilson, D. S., & Sober, E. (1989). Reviving the superorganism. *Journal of Theoretical Biology, 136,* 337–345.

14 "Mirror, Mirror, in My Mind": Empathy, Interpersonal Competence, and the Mirror Neuron System

Jennifer H. Pfeifer and Mirella Dapretto

During elementary school, children's report cards usually contain a section devoted to their "social skills," to provide parents with an idea of how well their child gets along with others, exhibits prosocial behavior, and displays appropriate emotional responses—including empathy—in interpersonal situations. Although the current political climate emphasizes academic success to the general neglect of social skills development, the systems underlying empathy and interpersonal competence remain a focus of continued research in the field of developmental, social, and clinical psychology, and more recently in the neurosciences as well. New directions are being forged by collaborations among these different disciplines. In this chapter we briefly discuss the multiple definitions of empathy across subfields and illustrate how these different characterizations of empathy have influenced research in the neurosciences. We then focus on a developmental definition of empathy and examine how this construct may be supported by a particular neural mechanism, the mirror neuron system (MNS). The potential role of the mirror neuron system in social developmental disorders, including autism, is also discussed. Finally, we outline future directions for a developmental social neuroscience approach to empathy.

Definitions of Empathy

Historically, as well as across disciplines, the definition of empathy has taken many forms (Preston & de Waal, 2002). A very early definition by Lipps (1903) depicted it as "feeling into" another individual's emotional state (*Einfühlung*). But what specific processes might underlie this "feeling into," and how are these processes instantiated in the typically developing and adult brain? Many suggest that empathy is a cognitive process of taking someone else's perspective, or imagining how that individual would feel in a particular situation (e.g., Deutsch & Maddle, 1975; Lamm, Batson, & Decety, 2007). Others point out that empathy, while being characterized as an emotional state that is isomorphic with that of another individual, also requires one to be consciously aware that the other individual is the source of the emotion in order to preclude self-focused distress and to foster other-oriented concern (e.g., de Vignemont & Singer, 2006; Gallup, 1982). These common definitions all contain some relatively explicit or intentional components—that is, they entail the volitional act of "putting oneself into somebody else's shoes." However, they also rely on a foundation of shared affect between self and other. This more basic aspect of empathy is frequently reflected in definitions taken from the developmental psychology literature. In that field, empathy is considered "an affective reaction that results from the apprehension or comprehension of another's emotional state or condition, and that is identical or very similar to what the other person is feeling or would be expected to feel" (Eisenberg & Fabes, 1998, p. 702), or "an affective response that is more appropriate to another's situation than one's own" (Hoffman, 2000, p. 4).

This experiential core of empathy—that is, the shared affect between self and other—is often associated with the construct of emotional contagion, wherein one's own emotional state results from the perception of another individual's emotion (Hatfield, Cacioppo, & Rapson, 1994) and from nonconscious behavioral mimicry of others' facial, vocal, and bodily expressions (also called the "chameleon effect"; Chartrand & Bargh, 1999). Emotional contagion and nonconscious mimicry help to coordinate behavior and emotions between interaction partners and may serve communicative functions (Bavelas et al., 1996). Significantly, individuals who show higher levels of spontaneous social imitation and affective resonance also score higher on scales assessing self-reported empathic behavior. These implicit processes also appear to increase liking and prosocial orientation (Chartrand & Bargh, 1999; van Baaren et al., 2004) as well as understanding of emotion (Niedenthal et al., 2001).

Interestingly, mimicry is also evident very early in development. Infants will imitate expressions and actions made by an experimenter within mere hours after birth (Meltzoff & Moore, 1977), and by six weeks they perform the more complicated task of imitating based on representations stored in memory (Meltzoff & Moore, 1994). Infants also cry in response to other infants' distress (Sagi & Hoffman, 1976). Does this mean that infants possess rudimentary empathic-like responses (or, as suggested by Dan Batson in chapter 1 of this volume, are babies who cry when another baby cries are simply competing for attention)? Meltzoff and colleagues have proposed that the imitative abilities of infants are supported by an innate system whereby seen actions (performed by others) are matched with felt actions (performed by oneself), allowing infants to map others' behavior onto their own mental representations and thus infer others' internal states through "analogy" to the self: "Infants imbue the acts of others with 'felt meaning,' because others are intrinsically recognized as 'like me'" (Meltzoff & Decety, 2003, p. 497). Although the evidence for this approach has been demonstrated primarily with regard to simple actions, it has been extended conceptually to account for the development of understanding others' intentions and emotions.

In a different vein, other developmental psychologists have been interested in the general relationship between empathy and interpersonal competence, so that, within this subfield, empathy can also be defined to some extent by the prosocial responses that it provokes (e.g., helping or expressions of concern; Eisenberg & Fabes, 1998; Eisenberg & Miller, 1987; Hoffman, 2000), or by the social dysfunction associated with its absence (e.g., autism spectrum disorder, psychopathy, sociopathy, and externalizing or other antisocial behaviors; Miller & Eisenberg, 1988; Preston & de Waal, 2002). From this perspective, it may be difficult to link empathy to the nonconscious mimicry and affect sharing observed in infants (Meltzoff & Moore, 1977; Sagi & Hoffman, 1976) because empathic behaviors—such as helping and concerned expressions—are first seen during the second year of life and are associated with increasing self-other differentiation and self-recognition (Zahn-Waxler et al., 1992; see also Lewis et al., 1989). Nevertheless, a focus on the emotional, affective aspects of empathy, as well as its relation to behavior and successful social interactions, dominates in the developmental psychology literature.

The emphasis on emotion and affect sharing, rather than cognition, in developmental approaches to empathy probably reflects the contribution of two factors. First, this emphasis helps to distinguish empathy from more general theory-of-mind abilities, because empathy is considered primarily an affective reaction involving a correspondence with others' emotions, rather than a cognitive process of reasoning about others' mental states (Premack & Woodruff, 1978; Wellman, 1991). Second, the latter developmental process is known to extend at least through the first decade of life, despite the frequent assertion that five-year-olds have attained a theory of mind (see Wellman & Liu, 2004). For example, conceptions of the mind as an active, independent agent are typically absent before ten years of age (Wellman & Hickling, 1994). Thus, one could hypothesize that the neural mechanisms supporting empathy might change with development, as children increasingly rely on conscious cognitive processes involving perspective taking as they refine their "mentalizing" abilities. In other words, being able to *feel* what others feel might be a phylogenetic and ontogenetic precursor to more explicit processes of *reasoning through* what others feel. As discussed previously, research suggests that automatic affective aspects of empathy, such as emotional contagion and affect sharing, are evident in infants and toddlers—significantly earlier than the explicit cognitive perspective-taking components of empathy, which are refined throughout the elementary school years (Hoffman, 2000; Litvack-Miller, McDougall, & Romney, 1997).

Neural Correlates of Empathy

Given the variety of ways empathy can be defined, probably the least controversial position to take is that empathy involves both affective and cognitive aspects. Affective component(s) may include some kind of shared feeling or emotional resonance, which may or may not be conscious. Importantly, this affective response might result in, result from, or be concurrent with cognitive component(s) of empathy, including explicit reasoning about another individual's emotional state as well as maintaining the distinction between oneself and others. In the past several years, neuroscience evidence for each of these components—cognitive perspective taking and distinguishing self from other, as well as shared affect—has elicited great interest in the research community.

Studies that examine the cognitive components of empathy typically compare imagining or observing emotional or painful situations (like being caught gossiping or receiving a painful shock) happening to oneself versus another individual. One region consistently active across these types of studies is the inferior parietal lobule (IPL), which is an area associated with multisensory integration. The laterality of activity there (stronger in the left hemisphere for self-perspectives and the right hemisphere for other-perspectives) might support the process of making self-other distinctions or attributing agency (Decety & Grèzes, 2006; Farrer et al., 2003; Lamm, Batson, & Decety, 2007; Ruby & Decety, 2003, 2004). Nearby, and somewhat difficult to distinguish in functional neuroimaging studies, is the temporoparietal junction (TPJ). Activity in the TPJ, particularly in the right hemisphere, has been associated with determining the contents of others' mental states (e.g., Saxe & Kanwisher, 2003; Saxe & Wexler, 2005). Two other brain regions frequently implicated in perspective-taking or mentalizing tasks include the temporal poles and medial prefrontal cortex (MPFC; Amodio & Frith, 2006). In addition to recruiting regions specifically involved in perspective taking, the brain might distinguish internal, personal experiences from external ones in two ways: (a) via the latency of the response—time-course data show that neural regions that produce similar responses to both perspectives still respond earlier when the experiences involve or are directed at the self instead of others; and (b) via the magnitude of the response—these regions also respond more intensely to self-perspectives than to other-perspectives (Decety & Grèzes, 2006).

Examining the neural correlates of perspective taking and self-other distinctions thus highlights ways in which the brain supports empathy through relatively explicit, cognitive means that are distinct from the processes supporting other kinds of social and nonsocial cognition. This approach parallels behavioral approaches in suggesting that mentalizing—reasoning about the mental states of others—is accomplished by naive psychology theories, which may be derived from innate domain-specific modules (Baron-Cohen, 1995; Leslie, 1987) or developed during childhood (Gopnik & Meltzoff, 1997; Wellman, 1991) but which, most importantly, are unique to thinking about other people (as opposed to animals, objects, and so on). An alternative approach conceives of mentalizing not in terms of special sets of rules and processes used to think about other individuals, but rather in terms of how the knowledge of one's own thoughts and feelings may be used to understand others via simulation, using the self as a model either implicitly (Gallese, 2006; Gallese & Goldman, 1998) or explicitly (Decety & Grèzes, 2006).

A host of neuroimaging studies have thus examined the patterns of activity that are common to a variety of emotional or affective situations experienced by the self or witnessed in others, typically focusing on the affective aspects of empathy. For example, shared networks in the anterior cingulate cortex (ACC) and anterior insula seem to be involved in both feeling pain and observing someone else experience pain (Botvinick et al., 2005;

Jackson et al., 2006; Jackson, Meltzoff, & Decety, 2005; Lamm, Batson, & Decety, 2007; Morrison et al. 2004; Saarela et al., 2006; Singer et al., 2004). Similarly, being disgusted oneself and observing others' disgust are both associated with activity in the anterior insula and adjacent areas of the inferior frontal gyrus (IFG) (Keysers & Gazzola, 2007; Wicker et al., 2003). Of central concern to this chapter is a specific network that has been proposed to encompass shared mental representation for actions in general (rather than specific emotions or affective experiences) regardless of their source: the mirror neuron system (MNS). We now turn to the MNS in greater detail.

The Mirror Neuron System and Emotion Understanding

The MNS was first described in the macaque brain, where neurons in ventral premotor cortex (area F5) and the inferior parietal lobule (area PF) fire either when the monkey executes goal-related hand actions or when it merely observes others (monkeys as well as humans) doing the same (Gallese et al., 1996; Rizzolatti et al., 1996). Although single-cell recordings cannot be readily obtained in humans, mirror-neuron-related responses in both the dorsal portion of the IFG (i.e., pars opercularis in putative Brodmann's area [BA] 44, the human homologue of area F5) and in the rostral portion of the IPL (i.e., the supramarginal gyrus in putative BA 40, the human homologue of area PF) have been demonstrated in humans using different neuroimaging techniques such as functional magnetic resonance imaging (fMRI; e.g., Iacoboni et al., 1999, 2005), transcranial magnetic stimulation (TMS; e.g., Fadiga, Craighero, & Olivier, 2005), and electroencephalography (EEG; e.g., Oberman, Pineda, & Ramachandran, 2007). The results of these studies highlight the important role of this system in understanding not only others' actions but their intentions and mental states as well (see Rizzolatti & Craighero, 2004, and Iacoboni & Dapretto, 2006, for reviews). Directly relevant to the neural underpinnings of empathy is the notion that the MNS may provide the neural mechanism by which we can understand others' emotions, a clear prerequisite for the ability to empathize with them. According to such models, further detailed below, the anterior portions of the insula play an important role in achieving an emotion representation by connecting the limbic system to mirror areas (Augustine, 1996; Carr et al., 2003).

The workings of this system provide a highly embodied perspective on how we come to understand others' emotions. In this view, the configuration of facial muscles denoting a particular emotional expression (e.g., furrowed eyebrows, scrunched-up nose, and pursed lips) is just another type of action associated with a motor plan that is activated—via the firing of mirror neurons in the pars opercularis—both when making an angry face and when observing an angry face in another individual. Through connections with the amygdala via the anterior insula, this action representation is in turn associated with an emotion representation: the feeling of anger. In other words, when I see your angry facial expression, that activates some of the same neural circuitry as when I myself am angry, allowing me to connect your action with the mental representation of anger—what this state means, what can elicit or alleviate it, and so on. Support for this model comes from studies demonstrating that both imitating and observing emotional expressions are associated with increased activity in the pars opercularis and the adjacent ventral premotor cortex, as well as in the insula and amygdala (Carr et al., 2003; Dapretto et al., 2006; Leslie, Johnson-Frey, & Grafton, 2004). In essence, the firing of mirror neurons during the observation of actions performed by another individual may code the equivalence between oneself and others. Once this mapping is achieved, an understanding of one's own emotions and intentions can be used to inform the understanding of others' behavior. The MNS may thus play an important role not only in the ability to empathize with others (Carr et al., 2003; Leslie, Johnson-Frey, & Grafton, 2004), but in social cognition and interpersonal competence in general (Gallese, Keysers, & Rizzolatti, 2004).

The Mirror Neuron System and Empathy

In our own work, we have seen strong evidence suggesting that the MNS may indeed be associated with the affective processes that support empathy (Pfeifer, Iacoboni, Mazziotta, & Dapretto, 2008). We elicited MNS activity by having 16 children (10 years of age; 7 girls) imitate or just observe various emotional expressions while undergoing two fMRI scans and we assessed children's self-reported tendency to empathize with others using a modified version of the Interpersonal Reactivity Index (IRI; Davis, 1983; Litvack-Miller, McDougall, & Romney, 1997). We found that children's self-reported ability to empathize was positively correlated with activity in both mirror neuron (pars opercularis in the IFG) and emotion representation (amygdala) regions during both the observation and imitation of emotional expressions ($t > 4.10$ for all maxima, $p < .05$ corrected for multiple comparisons at cluster level with a small-volume correction in the amygdala, rs (14) = .81 and .54 for the IFG and amygdala, respectively). The significant correlation between empathy and MNS activity suggests that internally mirroring the affective responses of others may constitute a mechanism that allows individuals to quite literally feel what others feel.

This study also shed some light on the neural correlates of different aspects of empathy. The IRI is composed of four subscales that assess distinct facets of interpersonal reactivity including empathic concern (the tendency to experience sympathy and related positive emotions oriented toward others), personal distress (the tendency to experience anxiety and related negative self-oriented emotions in empathy-arousing situations), fantasy (the degree to which one responds with empathy toward the emotions or actions of fictitious characters), and perspective taking (the tendency to adopt the point of view of another individual). Interestingly, we observed significant correlations between activity in mirror neuron and limbic regions and each of the first three subscales of the IRI (i.e., those tapping into the more affective components of empathy), but not with the perspective-taking subscale. In another recent study, right-lateralized MNS activity was also found to correlate with affective aspects of empathy (fantasy and empathic concern as assessed by the IRI) in adults (Kaplan & Iacoboni, 2006). However, perspective-taking abilities (as assessed by the IRI) were found to correlate with left-lateralized MNS activity in another study in adults (Gazzola, Aziz-Zadeh, & Keysers, 2006). Although the lack of a correlation between MNS activity and perspective-taking abilities in our developmental sample might reflect less developed mentalizing skills in children, the discrepancy between the two studies in adults suggests that the nature of the stimuli used to elicit mirror neuron activity may also influence the relationship observed between MNS activity and different aspects of empathy.

What about the role of the MNS in empathizing with others' pain? In a study examining the perception of pain from others' faces, positive correlations were found between various indicators of affect sharing (i.e., personal distress as measured by the IRI and empathic concern/interpersonal positivity as measured by the Balanced Emotional Empathy Scale (BEES); Mehrabian & Epstein, 1972) and activation in a cluster encompassing the anterior insula as well as the inferior frontal gyrus (although activity in this region encompassed the pars triangularis rather than the more dorsal pars opercularis; Saarela et al., 2006). Greater dispositional empathy, as assessed via the BEES and the empathic concern scale of the IRI, has also been associated with greater activation in the anterior insula and ACC, but not the pars opercularis, during the perception of a loved one's pain (Singer et al., 2004). However, in another recent study (Lamm, Batson, & Decety, 2007) relating neural activity associated with the observation of pain to several indices of dispositional empathy (IRI, Davis, 1983; Empathy Quotient, Baron-Cohen & Wheelwright, 2004; Emotional ZContagion Scale, Doherty, 1997; Emotion Regulation Scale, Gross & John, 2003), significant correlations were found between scores on the Emotional Contagion Scale and activity in both the frontal and parietal components of the MNS (though activity in these regions was attributed to their role in motor control rather than to mirroring mechanisms).

The limited MNS involvement found in these studies on pain, as compared to studies focusing on several different emotions (Carr et al., 2003; Dapretto et al., 2006; Leslie, Johnson-Frey, & Grafton, 2004) can be attributed to methodological differences. Both single-cell recordings in monkeys (e.g., Gallese et al., 1996) and neuroimaging data (e.g., Iacoboni et al., 1999) have clearly demonstrated that "mirror" responses (both neuronal firing and blood oxygen level–dependent [BOLD] activity) are weaker during action observation than during action execution. Furthermore, only a relatively small percentage of neurons (20% to 25%) that fire during action execution also fire during action observation (Rizzolatti & Craighero, 2004). Accordingly, mirror neuron-related activity may be hard to detect (i.e., it may not survive stringent statistical thresholds) in neuroimaging studies involving the repeated presentation of the same emotional expression, because the repetition leads to habituation and decreased BOLD responses (note, however, that suppression of BOLD activity with repeated stimulus presentation is actually a technique that can be used to identify the brain areas involved in a given task; Hamilton & Grafton, 2006).

The Mirror Neuron System and Interpersonal Competence

Taken together, the evidence presented above suggests that the MNS may support some aspects of empathy in both typically developing children and adults. But what about the hypothesis that the MNS may underlie more general social abilities (Gallese, Keysers, & Rizzolatti, 2004), and what about the emphasis in developmental psychology on the relationship between empathy and interpersonal competence (Eisenberg, 2000)? In our study relating MNS activity to empathy (described in the previous section), we also assessed children's social skills and behavior more generally using the Interpersonal Competence Scale (ICS; Cairns et al., 1995) in order to directly examine these relationships. Although the children's IRI and ICS scores were not significantly correlated with each other in our sample (r (14) = .32, ns), we found that the greater a child's interpersonal skills (as indexed by parental reports on the ICS), the greater the activity observed in the frontal component of the MNS (pars opercularis), as well as in the amygdala and anterior insula (whole-brain analyses, $t > 3.84$ for all maxima, $p < .05$ corrected for multiple comparisons at cluster level). This pattern of findings is fully consistent with the notion that the potentially automatic simulation mechanisms supported by the MNS—and its interface with the limbic system via the anterior insula—play a significant role in everyday social functioning (Gallese, Keysers, & Rizzolatti, 2004).

Further support for this hypothesis comes from a rapidly expanding literature indicating abnormal functioning of the MNS in autism, a developmental disorder characterized by marked impairments in the social domain. Indeed, evidence of MNS dysfunction in autism is remarkably consistent across studies conducted in different laboratories and using different techniques (for a review, see Oberman & Ramachandran, 2007). Using the same fMRI paradigm as in the study in typically developing children described above (Pfeifer et al., 2008), we examined MNS functioning in a sample of high-functioning children with autism spectrum disorder. Unlike what we observed in their normal controls (matched by age, gender, and IQ) as well as in our sample of typically developing children (Pfeifer et al., 2008), the imitation and observation of emotional expressions was not associated with significant MNS activity in the group of children with autism spectrum disorder, despite clear evidence they attended to the stimuli and performed the tasks just as well as children in the typically developing group (Dapretto et al., 2006). With regard to the role of the MNS in social cognition and behavior, we found that, at the individual level, MNS activity in children with autism spectrum disorder was strongly and negatively correlated with their level of social impairment as independently assessed by the children's scores on the social subscales of both the Autism Diagnostic Interview (Lord, Rutter, & Le Couteur, 1994) and the Autism Diagnostic Observational Schedule (Lord et al., 2000)—the gold-standard methods of autism assessment. In other words, to the degree that an autistic child exhibited less severe social deficits, there was incrementally more activity in the frontal component of the MNS (the pars opercularis in the IFG); conversely, the more severe the social impairments, the less the activity observed in MNS regions.

To our knowledge, the relationship between the MNS and interpersonal competence in normal individuals has been explored in only one other study (Lawrence et al., 2006), in which self-reported social skills (assessed via the Empathy Quotient; Baron-Cohen & Wheelwright, 2004) were positively associated with a small cluster of activity in the pars triangularis (adjacent to the pars opercularis) during a social perception task. In light of the existing controversy about the role of the MNS in social cognition (e.g., Saxe, 2005), future work in this area is clearly needed.

Conclusions and Future Directions

Taken together, the functional neuroimaging studies we have discussed provide rather convincing evidence that the human MNS is associated with individual differences in affective components of empathy—shared emotional states—as well as with more general social abilities. These associations appear to be especially prominent in children, in line with the notion that shared affect may provide a neural and behavioral foundation for interpersonal understanding. It is less clear what the role of the MNS may be with regard to more cognitive components of empathy, such as perspective taking. These more explicit aspects of empathy may or may not be related to MNS functioning, depending on whether the processes involve the use of information gathered via the MNS (e.g., I know you are feeling sad just by looking at you) or via other mechanisms (e.g., I know you are feeling sad because I heard your dog had to be put to sleep). The interplay between the more automatic form of empathizing afforded by the MNS and the more volitional empathizing afforded by explicit perspective taking should be explored in future studies if we are to fully understand the neural underpinnings of such a complex construct as empathy. Functional connectivity analyses or dynamic causal modeling techniques could prove useful in elucidating the roles played by the many "nodes" in the social brain network.

Another important query would ask what group or individual differences might affect MNS functioning in relation to empathy. For example, there may be gender differences such that females, on average, might exhibit stronger MNS involvement, as an evolutionary response to caretaking for the young. This would be consistent with the "extreme male brain" theory of autism (Baron-Cohen, 2002), which suggests that males on average are more analytical than empathic, whereas females exhibit the reverse pattern. Furthermore, in children and adults as well as in monkeys, behavioral empathy is known to increase with greater similarity between oneself and the target, on the basis of such factors as species, personality, age, or gender (for a review, see Preston & de Waal, 2002). Thus, while the basis of the interpersonal understanding achieved by the MNS is considered to be rooted within the self, features of one's interaction partner(s) may significantly impact mirroring processes. Indeed, there is some evidence that mirror neurons may possess sensitivities of this sort. One fMRI study showed greater MNS activity in response to the observation of actions performed by conspecifics (i.e., other humans) than actions by monkeys or dogs (Buccino et al., 2004). Gender might be the first meaningful social group to affect MNS functioning,

since (a) strong same-sex preferences for play partners develop at an early age and result in persistent gender segregation until puberty (e.g., Ruble & Martin, 1998), and (b) gender is also associated with differences in action/play styles (e.g., Maccoby & Jacklin, 1987), body type (Ruff, 2002), and facial structure (Ferrario et al., 1993).

Finally, from a developmental social neuroscience perspective, it is critical to look more closely at the relationship between empathy and other aspects of social cognitive development. For example, how does the development of emotion regulation relate to affective aspects of empathy and associated activity in mirror-neuron and limbic areas? How do emerging abilities to recognize the self or understand that others can possess diverse desires and beliefs affect the functioning of the MNS? And does the development of intergroup bias affect MNS responses to out-group members? Ultimately, a better understanding of the neural systems supporting both affective and cognitive components of empathy across development might help us design effective interventions for children diagnosed with pervasive social developmental disorders like autism, as well as training programs for the many typically developing children who are far from receiving top marks on the social skills section of their report card because they are lacking in empathy or related prosocial behaviors.

References

Amodio, D. M., & Frith, C. D. (2006). Meeting of minds: The medial frontal cortex and social cognition. *Nature Reviews Neuroscience, 7* (4), 268–277.

Augustine, J. R. (1996). Circuitry and functional aspects of the insular lobe in primates including humans. *Brain Research Reviews, 22*, 229–244.

Baron-Cohen, S. (1995). *Mindblindness: An essay on autism and theory of mind.* Cambridge, MA: MIT Press.

Baron-Cohen, S. (2002). The extreme male brain theory of autism. *Trends in Cognitive Sciences, 6* (6), 248–254.

Baron-Cohen, S., & Wheelwright, S. (2004). The empathy quotient: An investigation of adults with Asperger syndrome or high functioning autism, and normal sex differences. *Journal of Autism and Developmental Disorders, 34* (2), 163–175.

Bavelas, J. B., Black, A., Lemery, C. R., & Mullett, J. (1996). "I show you how you feel": Motor mimicry as a communicative act. *Journal of Personality and Social Psychology, 50*, 322–329.

Botvinick, M., Jha, A. P., Bylsma, L. M., Fabian, S. A., Solomon, P. E., & Prkachin, K. M. (2005). Viewing facial expressions of pain engages cortical areas involved in the direct experience of pain. *NeuroImage, 25*, 312–319.

Buccino, G., Vogt, S., Ritzl, A., Fink, G. R., Zilles, K., Freund, H. J., & Rizzolatti, G. (2004). Neural circuits underlying imitation learning of hand actions: An event-related fMRI study. *Neuron, 42* (2), 323–334.

Cairns, R. B., Leung, M.-C., Gest, S. D., & Cairns, B. D. (1995). A brief method for assessing social development: Structure, reliability, stability, and developmental validity of the interpersonal competence scale. *Behaviour Research and Therapy, 33,* 725–736.

Carr, L., Iacoboni, M., Dubeau, M. C., Mazziotta, J. C., & Lenzi, G. L. (2003). Neural mechanisms of empathy in humans: A relay from neural systems for imitation to limbic areas. *Proceedings of the National Academy of Sciences USA, 100* (9), 5497–5502.

Chartrand, T. L., & Bargh, J. A. (1999). The chameleon effect: The perception-behavior link and social interaction. *Journal of Personality and Social Psychology, 76* (6), 893–910.

Dapretto, M., Davies, M. S., Pfeifer, J. H., Scott, A. A., Sigman, M., Bookheimer, S. Y., et al. (2006). Understanding emotions in others: Mirror neuron dysfunction in children with autism spectrum disorders. *Nature Neuroscience, 9* (1), 28–30.

Davis, M. H. (1983). The effects of dispositional empathy on emotional reactions and helping: A multidimensional approach. *Journal of Personality, 51* (2), 167–184.

Decety, J., & Grèzes, J. (2006). The power of simulation: Imagining one's own and other's behavior. *Brain Research, 1079,* 4–14.

Deutsch, F., & Maddle, R. A. (1975). Empathy: Historic and current conceptualizations, measurement, and a cognitive theoretical perspective. *Human Development, 18,* 267–287.

De Vignemont, F., & Singer, T. (2006). The empathic brain: How, when and why? *Trends in Cognitive Sciences, 10* (10), 435–441.

Doherty, R.W. (1997). The emotional contagion scale: A measure of individual differences. *Journal of Nonverbal Behavior, 21,* 131-154.

Eisenberg, N. (2000). Emotion, regulation, and moral development. *Annual Review of Psychology, 51,* 665–697.

Eisenberg, N., & Fabes, R. A. (1998). Prosocial development. In W. Damon & N. Eisenberg (Eds.), *Handbook of child psychology* (pp. 701–778). New York: Wiley.

Eisenberg, N., & Miller, P. A. (1987). The relation of empathy to prosocial and related behaviors. *Psychological Bulletin, 101* (1), 91–119.

Fadiga, L., Craighero, L., & Olivier, E. (2005). Human motor cortex excitability during the perception of others' actions. *Current Opinion in Neurobiology, 15,* 213–218.

Farrer, C., Franck, N., Georgieff, N., Frith, C. D., Decety, J., & Jeannerod, M. (2003). Modulating the experience of agency: A positron emission tomography study. *NeuroImage, 18* (2), 324–333.

Ferrario, V. F., Sforza, C., Pizzini, G., Vogel, G., & Miani, A. (1993). Sexual dimorphism in the human face assessed by euclidean distance matrix analysis. *Journal of Anatomy, 183* (3), 593–600.

Gallese, V. (2006). Intentional attunement: A neurophysiological perspective on social cognition and its disruption in autism. *Brain Research, 1079* (1), 15–24.

Gallese, V., Fadiga, L., Fogassi, L., & Rizzolatti, G. (1996). Action recognition in the premotor cortex. *Brain, 119*, 593–609.

Gallese, V., & Goldman, A. I. (1998). Mirror neurons and the simulation theory of mind-reading. *Trends in Cognitive Sciences, 2* (12), 493–501.

Gallese, V., Keysers, C., & Rizzolatti, G. (2004). A unifying view of the basis of social cognition. *Trends in Cognitive Sciences, 8* (9), 396–403.

Gallup, G. G., Jr. (1982). Self-awareness and the emergence of mind in primates. *American Journal of Primatology, 2* (3), 237–248.

Gazzola, V., Aziz-Zadeh, L., & Keysers, C. (2006). Empathy and the somatotopic auditory mirror system in humans. *Current Biology, 16* (18), 1824–1829.

Gopnik, A., & Meltzoff, A. N. (1997). *Words, thoughts, and theories*. Cambridge, MA: MIT Press.

Gross, J. J., & John, O. P. (2003). Individual differences in two emotion regulation processes: Implications for affect, relationships, and well-being. *Journal of Personality and Social Psychology, 85*, 348–362.

Hamilton, A. F., & Grafton, S. T. (2006). Goal representation in human anterior intraparietal sulcus. *Journal of Neuroscience, 26* (4), 1133–1137.

Hatfield, E., Cacioppo, J. T., & Rapson, R. L. (1994). *Emotional contagion*. Paris: Cambridge University Press.

Hoffman, M. L. (2000). *Empathy and moral development: Implications for caring and justice*. New York: Cambridge University Press.

Iacoboni, M., & Dapretto, M. (2006). The mirror neuron system and the consequences of its dysfunction. *Nature Reviews Neuroscience, 7*, 942–951.

Iacoboni, M., Molnar-Szakacs, I., Gallese, V., Buccino, G., Mazziotta, J. C., & Rizzolatti, G. (2005). Grasping the intentions of others with one's mirror neuron system. *PLoS Biology, 3*, 529–535.

Iacoboni, M., Woods, R. P., Brass, M., Bekkering, H., Mazziotta, J. C., & Rizzolatti, G. (1999). Cortical mechanisms of human imitation. *Science, 286* (5449), 2526–2528.

Jackson, P. L., Brunet, E., Meltzoff, A. N., & Decety, J. (2006). Empathy examined through the neural mechanisms involved in imagining how I feel versus how you feel pain. *Neuropsychologia, 44* (5), 752–761.

Jackson, P. L., Meltzoff, A. N., & Decety, J. (2005). How do we perceive the pain of others? A window into the neural processes involved in empathy. *NeuroImage, 24* (3), 771–779.

Kaplan, J. T., & Iacoboni, M. (2006). Getting a grip on other minds: Mirror neurons, intention understanding and cognitive empathy. *Social Neuroscience, 1*, 175–183.

Keysers, C., & Gazzola, V. (2007). Integrating simulation and theory of mind: From self to social cognition. *Trends in Cognitive Sciences, 11*, 194–196.

Lamm, C., Batson, C. D., & Decety, J. (2007). The neural substrate of human empathy: Effects of perspective-taking and cognitive appraisal. *Journal of Cognitive Neuroscience, 19* (1), 42–58.

Lawrence, E. J., Shaw, P., Giampietro, V. P., Surguladze, S., Brammer, M. J., & David, A. S. (2006). The role of "shared representations" in social perception and empathy: An fMRI study. *NeuroImage, 29* (4), 1173–1184.

Leslie, A. (1987). Pretense and representation: The origins of a "theory of mind." *Psychological Review, 94*, 412–426.

Leslie, K. R., Johnson-Frey, S. H., & Grafton, S. T. (2004). Functional imaging of face and hand imitation: Towards a motor theory of empathy. *NeuroImage, 21* (2), 601–607.

Lewis, M., Sullivan, M. W., Stanger, C., & Weiss, M. (1989). Self development and self-conscious emotions. *Child Development, 60* (1), 146–156.

Lipps, T. (1903). Einfühlung, innere Nachahmung, und Organempfindungen. *Archiv für die gesamte Psychologie, 1*, 465–519.

Litvack-Miller, W., McDougall, D., & Romney, D. M. (1997). The structure of empathy during middle childhood and its relationship to prosocial behavior. *Genetic, Social, and General Psychology Monographs, 123* (3), 303–324.

Lord, C., Risi, S., Lambrecht, L., Cook, E. H., Jr., Leventhal, B. L., DiLavore, P. C., et al. (2000). The Autism Diagnostic Observation Schedule—Generic: A standard measure of social and communication deficits associated with the spectrum of autism. *Journal of Autism and Developmental Disorders, 30* (3), 205–223.

Lord, C., Rutter, M., & Le Couteur, A. (1994). Autism Diagnostic Interview—Revised: A revised version of a diagnostic interview for caregivers of individuals with possible pervasive developmental disorders. *Journal of Autism and Developmental Disorders, 24* (5), 659–685.

Maccoby, E. E., & Jacklin, C. N. (1987). Gender segregation in childhood. *Advances in Child Development and Behavior, 20*, 239–287.

Mehrabian, A., & Epstein, N. (1972). A measure of emotional empathy. *Journal of Personality, 40* (4), 525–543.

Meltzoff, A. N., & Decety, J. (2003). What imitation tells us about social cognition: A rapprochement between developmental psychology and cognitive neuroscience. *Philosophical Transactions of the Royal Society, London, B, 358*, 491–500.

Meltzoff, A. N., & Moore, M. K. (1977). Imitation of facial and manual gestures by human neonates. *Science, 198*, 74–78.

Meltzoff, A. N., & Moore, M. K. (1994). Imitation, memory, and the representation of persons. *Infant Behavior and Development, 17* (1), 83–99.

Miller, P. A., & Eisenberg, N. (1988). The relation of empathy to aggressive and externalizing/antisocial behavior. *Psychological Bulletin, 103* (3), 324–344.

Morrison, I., Lloyd, D., di Pellegrino, G., & Roberts, N. (2004). Vicarious responses to pain in anterior cingulate cortex: Is empathy a multisensory issue? *Cognitive, Affective, and Behavioral Neuroscience, 4* (2), 270–278.

Niedenthal, P. M., Brauer, M., Halberstadt, J. B., & Innes-Ker, A. H. (2001). When did her smile drop? Facial mimicry and the influences of emotional state on the detection of change in emotional expression. *Cognition and Emotion, 15* (6), 853–864.

Oberman, L. M., Pineda, J. A., & Ramachandran, V. S. (2007). The human mirror neuron system: a link between action observation and social skills. *Social, Cognitive, and Affective Neuroscience, 2,* 62–66.

Oberman, L. M., & Ramachandran, V. S. (2007). The simulating social mind: The role of the mirror neuron system and simulation in the social and communicative deficits of autism spectrum disorders. *Psychological Bulletin, 133* (2), 310–327.

Pfeifer, J. H., Iacoboni, M., Mazziotta, J. C., & Dapretto, M. (2008). Mirroring others' emotions relates to empathy and interpersonal competence in children. *NeuroImage, 39,* 2076–2085

Premack, D., & Woodruff, G. (1978). Chimpanzee problem-solving: A test for comprehension. *Science, 202* (4367), 532–535.

Preston, S. D., & de Waal, F. B. (2002). Empathy: Its ultimate and proximate bases. *Behavioral and Brain Sciences, 25* (1), 1–20; discussion 20–71.

Rizzolatti, G., & Craighero, L. (2004). The mirror-neuron system. *Annual Review of Neuroscience, 27,* 169–192.

Rizzolatti, G., Fadiga, L., Gallese, V., & Fogassi, L. (1996). Premotor cortex and the recognition of motor actions. *Cognitive Brain Research, 3* (2), 131–141.

Ruble, D. N., & Martin, C. L. (1998). Gender development. In W. Damon & N. Eisenberg (Eds.), *Handbook of child psychology* (pp. 933–1016). New York: Wiley.

Ruby, P., & Decety, J. (2003). What you believe versus what you think they believe: A neuroimaging study of conceptual perspective-taking. *European Journal of Neuroscience, 17* (11), 2475–2480.

Ruby, P., & Decety, J. (2004). How would you feel versus how do you think she would feel? A neuroimaging study of perspective-taking with social emotions. *Journal of Cognitive Neuroscience, 16* (6), 988–999.

Ruff, C. (2002). Variation in human body size and shape. *Annual Review of Anthropology, 31,* 211–232.

Saarela, M. V., Hlushchuk, Y., Williams, A. C., Schurmann, M., Kalso, E., & Hari, R. (2006). The compassionate brain: Humans detect intensity of pain from another's face. *Cerebral Cortex, 17,* 230-237.

Sagi, A., & Hoffman, M. L. (1976). Empathic distress in the newborn. *Developmental Psychology, 12,* 175–176.

Saxe, R. (2005). Against simulation: The argument from error. *Trends in Cognitive Sciences, 9,* 174–179.

Saxe, R., & Kanwisher, N. (2003). People thinking about thinking people. The role of the temporo-parietal junction in "theory of mind." *NeuroImage, 19* (4), 1835–1842.

Saxe, R., & Wexler, A. (2005). Making sense of another mind: The role of the right temporo-parietal junction. *Neuropsychologia, 43* (10), 1391–1399.

Singer, T., Seymour, B., O'Doherty, J., Kaube, H., Dolan, R. J., & Frith, C. D. (2004). Empathy for pain involves the affective but not sensory components of pain. *Science, 303*, 1157–1162.

Van Baaren, R. B., Holland, R. W., Kawakami, K., & van Knippenberg, A. (2004). Mimicry and prosocial behavior. *Psychological Science, 15* (1), 71–74.

Wellman, H. M. (1991). From desires to beliefs: Acquisition of a theory of mind. In A. Whiten (Ed.), *Natural theories of mind: Evolution, development and simulation of everyday mindreading* (pp. 19-38). Cambridge, MA: Blackwell.

Wellman, H. M., & Hickling, A. K. (1994). The mind's "I": Children's conceptions of the mind as an active agent. *Child Development, 65*, 1564–1580.

Wellman, H. M., & Liu, D. (2004). Scaling of theory-of-mind tasks. *Child Development, 75* (2), 523–541.

Wicker, B., Keysers, C., Plailly, J., Royet, J. P., Gallese, V., & Rizzolatti, G. (2003). Both of us disgusted in my insula: The common neural basis of seeing and feeling disgust. *Neuron, 40* (3), 655–664.

Zahn-Waxler, C., Radke-Yarrow, M., Wagner, E., & Chapman, M. (1992). Development of empathic concern for others. *Developmental Psychology, 28*, 126–136.

15   Empathy versus Personal Distress: Recent Evidence from Social Neuroscience

Jean Decety and Claus Lamm

Philosophers and social and developmental psychologists have long debated the nature of empathy (e.g., Batson et al., 1991; Eisenberg & Miller, 1987; Thompson, 2001) and whether the capacity to share and understand other people's emotions sets humans apart from other species (e.g., de Waal, 2005). Here, we consider empathy as a construct to account for a sense of similarity in feelings experienced by the self and the other without confusion between the two individuals (Decety & Jackson, 2004; Decety & Lamm, 2006). The experience of empathy can lead to sympathy (concern for another based on the apprehension or comprehension of the other's emotional state or condition), or even personal distress (i.e., an aversive, self-focused emotional reaction to the apprehension or comprehension of another's emotional state or condition) when there is confusion between self and other. Knowledge of empathic behavior is essential for an understanding of human social and moral development (Eisenberg et al., 1994). Furthermore, various psychopathologies are marked by empathy deficits, and a wide array of psychotherapeutic approaches stress the importance of clinical empathy as a fundamental component of treatment (Decety & Moriguchi, 2007; Farrow & Woodruff, 2007).

In recent years there has been an upsurge in neuroimaging investigations of empathy. Most of these studies reflect the new approach of social neuroscience, which combines research designs and behavioral measures used in social psychology with neurophysiological markers (Decety & Keenan, 2006). Such an approach plays an important role in disambiguating competing theories in social psychology in general and in empathy-related research in particular (Decety & Hodges, 2006). For instance, one critical question debated among social psychologists is whether perspective-taking instructions induce empathic concern and/or personal distress, and to what extent prosocial motivation springs from self-other overlap.

In this chapter we focus on recent social neuroscience research exploring how people respond behaviorally and neurally to the pain of others. The perception of others in painful situations constitutes an ecologically valid way to investigate the mechanisms underpinning the experience of empathy. Findings from these studies demonstrate that the mere perception of another individual in pain results, in the observer, in the activation of the neural network involved in the processing of firsthand experience of pain. This intimate overlap between the neural circuits responsible for our ability to perceive the pain of others and those underlying our own self-experience of pain supports the shared-representation theory of social cognition. This theory posits that perceiving someone else's emotion and having an emotional response, or subjective feeling state, both draw upon essentially the same computational processes and rely on somatosensory and motor representations. However, we argue that a complete self-other overlap can lead to personal distress and can possibly be detrimental to empathic concern. Personal distress may even result in a more egoistic motivation to reduce it, by withdrawing from the stressor, for example, thereby decreasing the likelihood of prosocial behavior (Tice, Bratslavsky, & Baumeister, 2001).

We first present the results of recent functional neuroimaging studies showing the involvement of shared neural circuits during the observation of pain in others and during the experience of pain in the self. Next, we discuss how perspective taking and the ability to differentiate the self from the other affect this sharing mechanism. In the final section, we examine how certain interpersonal variables modulate empathic concern and personal distress.

Shared Neural Circuits between Self and Other

It has long been suggested that empathy involves resonating with another person's unconscious affect. For instance, Basch (1983) speculated that, because conspecifics' respective autonomic nervous systems are genetically programmed to respond in a similar fashion, a given affective expression by a member of a particular species can trigger similar responses in other members of that species. The view that unconscious automatic mimicry of a target generates in the observer the autonomic response associated with that bodily state and facial expression subsequently received empirical support from a variety of behavioral and physiological studies. These studies investigated the perception-action coupling mechanism proposed by Preston and de Waal (2002). The core assumption of the perception-action model of empathy is that perceiving a target's state automatically activates the corresponding representations of that state in the observer, which in turn activates somatic and autonomic responses. The discovery of sensorimotor neurons (called mirror neurons) in the premotor and posterior parietal cortex that discharge during both the production of a given action and the perception of the same action performed by another individual provides the physiological mechanism for this direct link between perception and action (Rizzolatti & Craighero, 2004).

Behavioral studies demonstrate that viewing facial expressions triggers similar expressions on one's own face, even in the absence of conscious recognition of the stimulus. One functional magnetic resonance imaging (fMRI) experiment confirmed these results by showing that when participants were required to observe or to imitate facial expressions of various emotions, increased neurodynamic activity was detected in the brain regions implicated in the facial expressions of those emotions, including the superior temporal sulcus, the anterior insula, and the amygdala, as well as specific areas of the premotor cortex (Carr et al., 2003).

Accumulating evidence suggests that a "mirroring" or resonance mechanism is also at play both when one experiences sensory and affective feelings in the self and when one perceives them in others. Even at the level of the somatosensory cortex, seeing another's neck or face being touched elicits appropriately organized somatotopic activations in the brain of the observer (Blakemore et al., 2005). Robust support for the involvement of shared neural circuits in the perception of affective states comes from recent neuroimaging and transcranial magnetic stimulation (TMS) studies. For instance, the firsthand experience of disgust and the sight of disgusted facial expressions in others both activate the anterior insula (Wicker et al., 2003). Similarly, the observation of hand and face actions performed with an emotion engages regions that are also involved in the perception and experience of emotion and/or communication (Grosbras & Paus, 2006).

A number of neuroimaging studies recently demonstrated that the observation of pain in others recruits brain areas chiefly involved in the affective and motivational processing of direct pain perception (as illustrated in figure 15.1).

In one study, participants in the scanner received painful stimuli in some trials while in other trials they simply observed a signal indicating that their partner, who was present in the same room, would receive the painful stimuli (Singer et al., 2004). During both types of trials the medial and anterior cingulate cortex (MCC and ACC) and the anterior insula were activated (see also Morrison et al., 2004). These regions contribute to the affective and motivational processing of noxious stimuli, the aspects of pain processing that pertain to desires, urges, or impulses to avoid or terminate a painful experience. Similar results were reported in a study by Jackson, Meltzoff, and Decety (2005) in which participants were shown pictures of people's hands or feet in painful situations or in neutral everyday-life situations. Significant activation in regions involved in the affective aspects of pain processing (MCC, ACC, and anterior insula) was detected but, as in the study by Singer and colleagues (2004), no signal change was found in the somatosensory cortex. However, a recent TMS study did report changes in corticospinal motor representations of hand muscles in individuals observing needles penetrating the hands or feet of a human model (Avenanti et al., 2005), indicating that the observation of pain can also involve sensorimotor representations.

In summary, current neuroscientific evidence suggests that merely observing another individual in a painful situation yields responses in the neural network associated with the coding of the motivational-affective dimension of pain in oneself. On the other hand, a recent meta-analysis of neuroimaging studies indicates that this overlap is not complete (Jackson, Rainville, & Decety, 2006). Both in the insula and in the cingulate cortex, the perception of pain in others results in more rostral activations than does the firsthand experience of pain. Also, vicariously instigated activations in the pain matrix are not

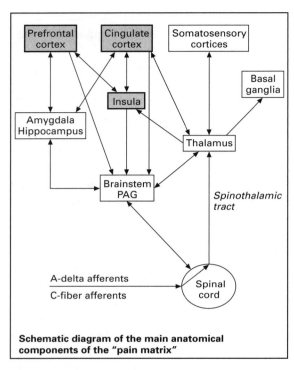

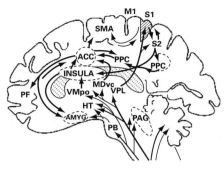

→ **The primary (S1) and secondary (S2) sensory cortices** are involved in the sensory-discriminative aspects of pain, e.g., the bodily location and intensity of the stimulus.

→ **ACC and insula** subserve the affective-motivational component, i.e., the evaluation of subjective discomfort and response preparation in the context of painful or aversive stimuli.

Schematic diagram of the main anatomical components of the "pain matrix"

Figure 15.1
Neurophysiological research on pain points to a distinction between the sensory-discriminative aspect of pain processing and the affective-motivational one. These two aspects are underpinned by discrete yet interacting neural networks.

necessarily specific to the emotional experience of pain; they may be shared by other processes such as somatic monitoring, negative stimulus evaluation, and the selection of appropriate skeletomuscular movements of aversion. Thus, the shared neural representations in the affective-motivational part of the pain matrix might not be specific to the sensory qualities of pain, but instead be associated with more general survival mechanisms such as aversion and withdrawal.

The discovery that the observation of pain in others activates brain structures involved in negative emotional experiences has important implications for the question of whether observing another's plight will result in empathic concern or personal distress. Appraisal theory views emotions as resulting from the appraisal of physiological responses triggered by an external or internal stimulus (Scherer, Schorr, & Johnstone, 2001). Perceiving the emotions of others is a powerful instigator of physiological responses, leading to distinct changes in both the central and the autonomic nervous system. Interestingly, a higher linkage between observer and target in psychophysiological indicators such as heart rate and electrodermal activity predicts better understanding of the target's emotional state (Levenson & Ruef, 1992). Note also that parts of the insula and the MCC that are active during the observation of pain in others contribute to the monitoring of bodily changes, such as visceral and somatic responses. Hence it is plausible that, depending upon whether these responses are attributed to the self or to the other, they might result in more or less other- versus self-oriented emotions.

Perspective Taking, Self-Other Awareness, and Empathy

There is general consensus among theorists that the ability to adopt and entertain the psychological perspective of others has a number of important consequences. Well-developed perspective-taking abilities allow us to overcome our usual egocentrism and tailor our behaviors to others' expectations (Davis et al., 1996). Further, successful role taking has been linked to moral reasoning and altruism (Batson et al., 1991). Using mental imagery to take the perspective of another is a powerful way to place oneself in the situation or emotional state of that person. Mental imagery not only enables us to see the world of our conspecifics through their eyes or as if in their shoes, but may also result in similar sensations as the other person's (Decety & Grèzes, 2006).

Social psychologists have for a long time been interested in the distinction between imagining the other and imagining oneself, and in particular in the emotional and motivational consequences of these two perspectives. A number of relevant studies show that focusing on another's feelings (imagining the other) may evoke stronger empathic concern, while explicitly putting oneself into the shoes of the target (imagining the self) induces both empathic concern and personal distress. In one such study, Batson, Early, and Salvarini (1997) investigated the affective consequences of different perspective-taking instructions when participants listened to a story about Katie Banks, a young college student struggling with her life after the death of her parents. This study showed that different instructions had distinct effects on how participants perceived the target's situation. Notably, participants who imagined themselves to be in Katie's place showed stronger signs of discomfort and personal distress than participants who focused on the target's responses and feelings (imagine other) or those who were instructed to take on an objective, detached point of view. In addition, both imagine-other and imagine-self conditions differed from the detached perspective by promoting greater empathic concern. This outcome may help to explain why observing a need situation does not always result in prosocial behavior: if perceiving another person in an emotionally or physically painful circumstance elicits personal distress, the observer may tend not to fully attend to the other's experience, and as a result may fail to display sympathetic behaviors.

Cognitive neuroscience research demonstrates that when individuals adopt the perspective of others, neural circuits common to the ones underlying first-person experiences are activated as well. However, taking the perspective of the other produces additional activation in specific parts of the frontal cortex that are implicated in executive functions, particularly inhibitory control (e.g., Ruby & Decety, 2003, 2004). In line with these findings, the frontal lobes may functionally serve to separate perspectives, helping one to resist interference from one's own perspective when adopting the subjective perspective of another (Decety & Jackson, 2004). This ability is of particular importance when observing another's distress, because a complete merging with the target would lead to confusion as to who is experiencing the negative emotions and therefore to different motivations as to who should be the target of supportive behavior.

In two successive functional MRI studies, we recently investigated the neural mechanisms subserving the effects of perspective taking during the perception of pain in others. In the first study, participants were shown pictures of hands and feet in painful situations and asked to either imagine themselves or to imagine another individual experiencing these situations and rate the level of pain the situations would induce (Jackson, Brunet, et al., 2006). Both the self-perspective and the other-perspective were associated with activation in the neural network involved in pain processing. This finding is consistent with the account of social perception as a function of shared neural representations, discussed above. However, the self-perspective yielded higher pain ratings and quicker response times, and the involvement of the pain matrix was more extensive in the secondary somatosensory cortex, a subarea of the MCC, and the insula.

In a second neuroimaging study, the distinction between empathic concern and personal distress was investigated in more detail using a number of additional behavioral measures and a set of ecological and extensively validated dynamic stimuli (Lamm, Batson, & Decety, 2007). Participants watched a series of video clips featuring patients undergoing painful medical treatment. They were asked to either put themselves explicitly in the shoes of the patient (imagine self), or to focus on the patients' feelings and affective expressions (imagine other). The behavioral data confirmed that explicitly projecting oneself into an aversive situation leads to higher personal distress, whereas focusing on the emotional and behavioral reactions of another to the same plight is accompanied by higher empathic concern and lower personal distress (see figure 15.2). The neuroimaging data were consistent with this finding and provided some insights into the neural correlates of these distinct behavioral responses. The self-perspective evoked stronger hemodynamic responses in brain regions involved in coding the motivational-affective dimensions of pain, including the bilateral insular cortices, the anterior MCC, the amygdala, and various structures involved in action control. The amygdala plays a critical role in fear-related behaviors, such as the evaluation of actual or potential threats. Imagining oneself to be in a painful and potentially dangerous situation might therefore have triggered a stronger fearful or aversive response than imagining someone else to be in the same situation.

In keeping with findings by Jackson, Brunet, and colleagues (2006), this insular activation was also located in a more posterior, middorsal subsection of the area. The middorsal part

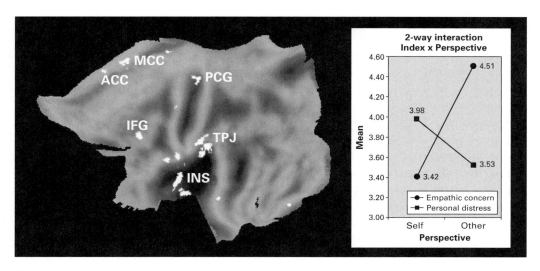

Figure 15.2
Neural and behavioral consequences of two different perspective-taking instructions (adapted from Lamm, Batson, & Decety, 2007). The flat-map representation of the left hemisphere shows higher activations during the self-perspective in limbic/paralimbic (medial and anterior cingulate cortex [MCC and ACC], insula [INS]) and cortical brain structures (temporoparietal junction [TPJ], inferior frontal gyrus [IFG], postcentral gyrus [PCG]). The overlay of functional activation on the flattened cortical surface was created using Caret (http://brainmap.wustl.edu/caret) and Van Essen et al., 2001.

of the insula plays a role in coding the sensorimotor aspects of painful stimulation, and it has strong connections with the basal ganglia, where activity was also higher during the self-perspective. Taken together, these considerations suggest that the insular activity generated in the self-perspective reflects simulation of sensory aspects of the painful experience. Such a simulation might serve to mobilize motor areas in preparation for defensive or withdrawal behaviors and also to instigate the interoceptive monitoring associated with the autonomic changes that the simulation process evokes (Critchley et al., 2005). Such an interpretation also accounts for the activation difference present in the somatosensory cortex. Finally, the higher activation in premotor structures might connect with a stronger mobilization of motor representations by the more stressful and discomforting first-person perspective. Further support for this interpretation is provided by the results of a positron emission tomography study that investigated the relationship between situational empathic accuracy and brain activity, which also found higher activation in medial premotor structures, partially extending into the MCC, when participants witnessed the distress of others (Shamay-Tsoory et al., 2005). That study also pointed to the importance of prefrontal areas in the understanding of distress.

Taken together, the available empirical findings reveal important differences in the neural systems involved in first- and third-person perspective taking, and they contradict the notion that the self and other completely merge in the experience of empathy. The specific activation differences in both the affective and sensorimotor aspects of the pain matrix, along with the higher pain and distress ratings, seem to reflect the self-perspective's requirement of more direct and personal involvement. One key region that might facilitate self-versus-other distinctions is the right temporoparietal junction (TPJ). The TPJ is activated in most neuroimaging studies of empathy (Decety & Lamm, 2007), and it seems to play a decisive role in self-awareness and the sense of agency. Agency (i.e., the awareness of oneself as the initiator of actions, desires, thoughts, and feelings) is essential for successful navigation of shared representations between self and other (Decety, 2005; Decety & Lamm, 2007).

Thus, self-awareness and a sense of agency both play pivotal roles in empathy and significantly contribute to social interaction. These capacities are likely to be involved in distinguishing emotional contagion—which relies heavily on the automatic link between perceiving the emotions of another and one's own experience of the same emotion—from empathic responses, which call for a more detached relation. The neural responses that have been found not to overlap between the self and other perspectives may take advantage of available processing capacities to plan appropriate future actions concerning the other. Awareness of our own feelings, and the ability to consciously regulate our own emotions, may allow us to disconnect empathic responses to others from our own personal distress, such that only the former leads to prosocial behavior.

Modulation of Empathic Responding

The mere perception of the behavior of others activates corresponding circuits in the self, and the perception of others' painful situations activates neural circuits involved in the firsthand experience of pain. But there is also evidence that this unconscious empathic responding can be modulated by various situational and dispositional variables. Research in social psychology has identified a number of these factors, such as the relationship between the target and the empathizer, the empathizer's dispositions, and the context in which the social interaction takes place. Accordingly, whether observing the distress of a close friend results in empathic concern and helping behavior or in withdrawal from the situation depends on the complex interaction of all these factors.

Emotion regulation seems to have a particularly important role in social interaction, and it has a clear adaptive function for both the individual and the species (Ochsner & Gross, 2005). Of note, it has been demonstrated that individuals who can regulate their emotions are more likely to experience empathy and to interact in morally desirable ways with others (Eisenberg et al., 1994). In contrast, people who experience their emotions intensely, especially negative emotions, are more prone to personal distress, an aversive emotional reaction (e.g., anxiety or discomfort) that is based on the recognition of another's emotional state or condition.

In the case of perception of others in pain, the ability to down-regulate one's emotions is particularly valuable when the distress of the target becomes overwhelming. For example, a mother alarmed by her baby's cries at night has to cope with her own discomfort in order to provide appropriate care for her distressed offspring. One strategy to regulate one's emotions is based on cognitive reappraisal. This involves reinterpreting the valence of a stimulus in order to change the way in which we respond to it. Such reappraisal can be achieved intentionally, or it can result from the processing of additional information about the emotion-eliciting stimulus.

In the fMRI study mentioned above in which participants watched videos of painful medical treatment, Lamm, Batson, and Decety (2007) investigated the effects of cognitive appraisal on the experience of empathy by providing differing information about the consequences of the observed pain. The observed target patients belonged to two different groups. In one group, health and quality of life improved after the painful therapy, while members of the other group did not benefit from the treatment. Thus, stimuli of identically arousing and negatively valenced emotional content were watched, but the participants were given different contexts in which to appraise the patients' pain. The results confirmed the authors' hypotheses and demonstrated that one's appraisal of an aversive event can considerably alter one's responses to it. Patients undergoing noneffective treatment were judged to experience higher levels of pain, and personal distress in the observers was more pronounced when watching videos of those patients. Brain activation was modulated in two subregions of the orbitofrontal cortex (OFC) and in the rostral part of the MCC. The OFC is known to play an important role in the evaluation of positive and negative reinforcements and is also involved in emotion reappraisal. Activity in the OFC may thus reflect evaluation of the valence of presented stimuli. Interestingly, watching effectively versus noneffectively treated patients did not modulate the hemodynamic activity in either the visual-sensory areas or the insula. This suggests that both patient groups triggered an emotional reaction and that top-down mechanisms did not alter stimulus processing at an early perceptual stage.

Another intrapersonal factor affecting the empathic response is the emotional background state of the observer (Niedenthal et al., 2000). For example, a depressive mood can affect the way in which we perceive the expression of emotions by others. In a recent developmental neuroscience study, limbic structures such as the amygdala and the nucleus accumbens became hyperactive when participants with pediatric bipolar disorder attended to the facial expression of emotion (Pavuluri et al., 2008). Similarly, patients with generalized social phobia showed increased amygdala activation when exposed to angry or contemptuous faces (Stein et al., 2002).

Whether individual differences in dispositional empathy and personal distress modulate the occurrence and intensity of self- versus other-centered responding is currently a matter of debate. Several recent neuroimaging studies demonstrate specific relationships between brain activity and questionnaire measures of empathy. For example, both Singer and colleagues (2004) and Lamm and colleagues (2007) detected significantly increased activation in insular and cingulate cortices in participants with higher self-reported empathy during perception. These findings showed modulation of neural activity in the very brain regions that are involved in coding the affective response to the other's distress. Note however, that no such correlations were found in a similar study (Jackson, Meltzoff, & Decety, 2005). Also, no correlations with self-report personal distress scores were observed by Lamm, Batson, and Decety (2007) or by Jackson, Brunet, and their coworkers (2006). However, Lawrence and colleagues (2006) did report such correlations with activity in the cingulate and prefrontal regions of participants who labeled a target's mental and affective state. Part of the discrepancy between the neuroscience research and the dispositional measures may be related to the low validity of self-report measures in predicting actual empathic behavior (Davis & Kraus, 1997; Ickes, 2003). It is our conviction that brain-behavior correlations should be treated with caution, and that care must be taken to formulate specific hypotheses both about the neural correlates of the dispositional measures and about what the questionnaire actually measures. For example, scores on the personal distress subscale of the Interpersonal Reactivity Index (Davis, 1996) yielded correlations close to zero with the experimentally derived distress measures, and no significant correlations with brain activation. This outcome indicates that the subscale is probably not an appropriate measure of situative discomfort evoked by the observation of another's distress.

The effects of *interpersonal* factors—such as the similarity or closeness between the empathizer and the target—have been investigated at the behavioral, psychophysiological, and neural levels. For instance, Cialdini and coworkers (1997) have documented that perceived oneness—the perceived overlap between self and other—is an important predictor of helping behavior and correlates strongly with empathic concern. Lanzetta and Englis (1989) made interesting observations concerning the effects of attitudes on social interaction. Their studies show that, in a competitive relationship, observation of the other's joy results in distress, whereas pain in the competitor leads to positive emotions. These findings reflect an important and often ignored aspect of empathy, namely that the ability can also be used in a malevolent way, as when knowledge about the emotional or cognitive state of competitors is used to harm them. A recent study by Singer and colleagues (2006) revealed the neural correlates of such counterempathic responding. In that study, participants were first engaged in a sequential prisoner's dilemma game with confederate targets who were playing the game either fairly or unfairly. Following this behavioral manipulation, fMRI measures were taken during the observation of fair and unfair players receiving painful stimulation. Compared to the observation of fair players, participants' observation of unfair players in pain led to significantly reduced activation in brain areas coding the affective components of pain. This effect, however, was detected in male participants only, who also exhibited a concurrent increase of activation in reward-related areas.

In sum, there is strong behavioral evidence demonstrating that the experience of empathy and personal distress can be modulated by a number of social and cognitive factors. In addition, a few recent neuroscience studies indicate that such modulation leads to activity changes in the neural systems that process social information. Further studies are required to increase our knowledge about the various factors, processes, and (neural and behavioral) effects involved in and resulting from the modulation of empathic responses. This knowledge will inform us about how empathy can be channeled into prosocial and altruistic behaviors.

Conclusion

The combined results of functional neuroimaging studies demonstrate that when individuals perceive others in pain or distressful situations, they use the same neural mechanisms as when they are in painful situations themselves. Such a shared neural mechanism offers an interesting foundation for intersubjectivity because it provides a functional bridge between first-person information and third person information, grounded in self-other equivalence (Decety & Sommerville, 2003; Sommerville & Decety, 2006), that allows analogical reasoning and offers a possible route to understanding others. Yet a minimal distinction between self and other is essential for social interaction in general and for empathy in particular, and new work in social neuroscience has demonstrated that the self and other are distinguished at both the behavioral and neural levels. Finally, recent cognitive neuroscience research indicates that the neural response to others in pain can be modulated by various situational and dispositional variables.

Taken together, these data support the view that empathy operates by way of conscious and automatic processes that, far from functioning independently, represent different aspects of a common mechanism. These accounts of empathy are in harmony with theories of embodied cognition, which contend that cognitive representations and operations are fundamentally grounded in bodily states and in the brain's modality-specific systems (Niedenthal et al., 2005).

Acknowledgment

The writing of this chapter was supported by a National Science Foundation grant (BCS 0718480) to Jean Decety.

References

Avenanti, A., Bueti, D., Galati, G., & Aglioti, S. M. (2005). Transcranial magnetic stimulation highlights the sensorimotor side of empathy for pain. *Nature Neuroscience 8*, 955–960.

Basch, M. F. (1983). Empathic understanding: A review of the concept and some theoretical considerations. *Journal of the American Psychoanalytic Association, 31,* 101–126.

Batson, C. D., Batson, J. G., Singlsby, J. K., Harrell, K. L., Peekna, H. M., & Todd, R. M. (1991). Empathic joy and the empathy-altruism hypothesis. *Journal of Personality and Social Psychology, 61,* 413–426.

Batson, C. D., Early, S., & Salvarini, G. (1997). Perspective taking: Imagining how another feels versus imagining how you would feel. *Personality and Social Personality Bulletin, 23,* 751–758.

Blakemore, S. J., Bristow, D., Bird, G., Frith, C., & Ward, J. (2005). Somatosensory activations during the observation of touch and a case of vision-touch synaesthesia. *Brain 128,* 1571–1583.

Carr, L., Iacoboni, M., Dubeau, M. C., Mazziotta, J. C., & Lenzi, G. L. (2003). Neural mechanisms of empathy in humans: A relay from neural systems for imitation to limbic areas. *Proceedings of the National Academy of Sciences USA, 100,* 5497–5502.

Cialdini, R. B., Brown, S. L., Lewis, B. P., Luce, C., & Neuberg, S. L. (1997). Reinterpreting the empathy-altruism relationship: When one into one equals oneness. *Journal of Personality and Social Psychology, 73,* 481–494.

Critchley, H. D., Wiens, S., Rotshtein, P., Öhman, A., & Dolan, R. D. (2005). Neural systems supporting interoceptive awareness. *Nature Neuroscience, 7,* 189–195.

Davis, M. H., Conklin, L., Smith, A., & Luce, C. (1996). Effect of perspective taking on the cognitive representation of persons: A merging of self and other. *Journal of Personality and Social Psychology, 70,* 713–726.

Davis, M. H. (1996). *Empathy: A social psychological approach.* Madison, WI: Westview Press.

Davis, M. H., & Kraus, L. A. (1997). Personality and empathic accuracy. In W. Ickes (Ed.), *Empathic accuracy* (pp. 144–168). New York: Guilford Press.

Decety, J. (2005). Perspective taking as the royal avenue to empathy. In B. F. Malle and S. D. Hodges (Eds.), *Other minds: How humans bridge the divide between self and other* (pp. 135–149). New York: Guilford Press.

Decety, J., & Grèzes, J. (2006). The power of simulation: Imagining one's own and other's behavior. *Brain Research, 1079,* 4–14.

Decety, J., & Hodges, S. D. (2006). A social cognitive neuroscience model of human empathy. In P. A. M. van Lange (Ed.), *Bridging social psychology: Benefits of transdisciplinary approaches* (pp. 103–109). Mahwah, NJ: Erlbaum.

Decety, J., & Jackson, P. L. (2004). The functional architecture of human empathy. *Behavioral and Cognitive Neuroscience Reviews, 3,* 71–100.

Decety, J., & Keenan, J. P. (2006). Social neuroscience: A new journal. *Social Neuroscience, 1,* 1–4.

Decety, J., & Lamm, C. (2006). Human empathy through the lens of social neuroscience. *Scientific World Journal, 6,* 1146–1163.

Decety, J., & Lamm, C. (2007). The role of the right temporoparietal junction in social interaction: How low-level computational processes contribute to meta-cognition. *Neuroscientist, 13,* 580–593.

Decety, J., & Moriguchi, Y. (2007). The empathic brain and its dysfunction in psychiatric populations: Implications for intervention across different clinical conditions. *BioPsychoSocial Medicine, 1,* 22–65.

Decety, J., & Sommerville, J. A. (2003). Shared representations between self and others: A social cognitive neuroscience view. *Trends in Cognitive Sciences, 7,* 527–533.

De Waal, F. (2005). Primates, monks and the mind. *Journal of Consciousness Studies, 12,* 1–17.

Eisenberg, N., Fabes, R. A., Murphy, B., Karbon, M., Maszk, P., Smith, M., O'Boyle, C., & Suh, K. (1994). The relations of emotionality and regulation to dispositional and situational empathy-related responding. *Journal of Personality and Social Psychology, 66,* 776–797.

Eisenberg, N., & Miller, P. A. (1987). The relation of empathy to prosocial and related behaviors. *Psychological Bulletin, 101,* 91–119.

Farrow, T., & Woodruff, P. W. (2007). *Empathy in mental illness and health.* Cambridge: Cambridge University Press.

Grosbras, M. H., & Paus, T. (2006). Brain networks involved in viewing angry hands or faces. *Cerebral Cortex, 16,* 1087–1096.

Ickes, W. (2003). *Everyday mind reading: Understanding what other people think and feel.* Amherst, NY: Prometheus Books.

Jackson, P. L., Brunet, E., Meltzoff, A. N., & Decety, J. (2006). Empathy examined through the neural mechanisms involved in imagining how I feel versus how you feel pain. *Neuropsychologia, 44,* 752–761.

Jackson, P. L., Meltzoff, A. N., & Decety, J. (2005). How do we perceive the pain of others? A window into the neural processes involved in empathy. *NeuroImage, 24,* 771–779.

Jackson, P. L., Rainville, P., & Decety, J. (2006). From nociception to empathy: The neural mechanism for the representation of pain in self and in others. *Pain, 125,* 5–9.

Lamm, C., Batson, C. D., & Decety, J. (2007). The neural basis of human empathy: Effects of perspective-taking and cognitive appraisal. *Journal of Cognitive Neuroscience, 19,* 42–58.

Lanzetta, J. T., & Englis, B. G. (1989). Expectations of cooperation and competition and their effects on observers' vicarious emotional responses. *Journal of Personality and Social Psychology, 56,* 543–554.

Lawrence, E. J., Shaw, P., Giampietro, V. P., Surguladze, S., Brammer, M. J., & David, A. S. (2006). The role of "shared representations" in social perception and empathy: An fMRI study. *NeuroImage, 29,* 1173–1184.

Levenson, R. W., & Ruef, A. M. (1992). Empathy: A physiological substrate. *Journal of Personality and Social Psychology, 63,* 234–246.

Morrison, I., Lloyd, D., di Pellegrino, G., & Roberts, N. (2004). Vicarious responses to pain in anterior cingulate cortex: Is empathy a multisensory issue? *Cognitive and Affective Behavioral Neuroscience, 4,* 270–278.

Niedenthal, P. M., Barsalou, L. W., Ric, F., & Krauth-Gruber, S. (2005). Embodiment in the acquisition and use of emotion knowledge. In L. Feldman Barrett, P. M. Niedenthal, & P. Winkielman (Eds.), *Emotions and consciousness* (pp. 21–50). New York: Guilford Press.

Niedenthal, P. M., Halberstadt, J. B., Margolin, J., & Innes-Ker, A. H. (2000). Emotional state and the detection of change in the facial expression of emotion. *European Journal of Social Psychology, 30,* 211–222.

Ochsner, K. N., & Gross, J. J. (2005). The cognitive control of emotion. *Trends in Cognitive Sciences, 9,* 242–249.

Pavuluri, M. N., O'Connor, M. M., Harral, E., & Sweeney, J. A. (2008). Affective neural circuitry during facial emotion processing in pediatric bipolar disorder. *Biological Psychiatry, 162,* 244–255.

Preston, S. D., & de Waal, F. B. M. (2002). Empathy: Its ultimate and proximate bases. *Behavioral Brain Science, 25,* 1–72.

Rizzolatti, G., & Craighero, L. (2004). The mirror-neuron system. *Annual Review in Neuroscience, 27,* 169–192.

Ruby, P., & Decety, J. (2003). What you believe versus what you think they believe? A neuroimaging study of conceptual perspective taking. *European Journal of Neuroscience, 17,* 2475–2480.

Ruby, P., & Decety, J. (2004). How would you feel versus how do you think she would feel? A neuroimaging study of perspective taking with social emotions. *Journal of Cognitive Neuroscience, 16,* 988–999.

Scherer, K. R., Schorr, A., & Johnstone, T. (2001). *Appraisal processes in emotion.* New York: Oxford University Press.

Shamay-Tsoory, S. G., Lester, H., Chisin, R., Israel, O., Bar-Shalom, R., Peretz, A., Tomer, R., Tsitrinbaum, Z., & Aharon-Peretz, J. (2005). The neural correlates of understanding the other's distress: A positron emission tomography investigation of accurate empathy. *NeuroImage, 15,* 468–472.

Singer, T., Seymour, B., O'Doherty, J., Kaube, H., Dolan, R. J., & Frith, C. D. (2004). Empathy for pain involves the affective but not the sensory components of pain. *Science, 303,* 1157–1161.

Singer, T., Seymour, B., O'Doherty, J. P., Stephan, K. E., Dolan, R. J., & Frith, C. D. (2006). Empathic neural responses are modulated by the perceived fairness of others. *Nature, 439,* 466–469.

Sommerville, J. A., & Decety, J. (2006). Weaving the fabric of social interaction: Articulating developmental psychology and cognitive neuroscience in the domain of motor cognition. *Psychonomic Bulletin and Review, 13* (2), 179–200.

Stein, M. B., Goldin, P. R., Sareen, J., Zorrilla, L. T., & Brown, G. G. (2002). Increased amygdala activation to angry and contemptuous faces in generalized social phobia. *Archives of General Psychiatry, 59,* 1027–1034.

Thompson, E. (2001). Empathy and consciousness. *Journal of Consciousness Studies, 8,* 1–32.

Tice, D. M., Bratslavsky, E., & Baumeister, R. F. (2001). Emotional distress regulation takes precedence over impulse control: If you feel bad, do it! *Journal of Personality and Social Psychology, 80,* 53–67.

Van Essen, D. C., Dickson, J., Harwell, J., Hanlon, D., Anderson, C. H., & Drury, H. A. (2001). An integrated software system for surface-based analyses of cerebral cortex. *Journal of the American Medical Informatics Association, 41,* 1359–1378.

Wicker, B., Keysers, C., Plailly, J., Royet, J. P., Gallese, V., & Rizzolatti, G. (2003). Both of us disgusted in my insula: The common neural basis of seeing and feeling disgust. *Neuron, 40,* 655–664.

16 Empathic Processing: Its Cognitive and Affective Dimensions and Neuroanatomical Basis

Simone G. Shamay-Tsoory

Empathy is a central concept in psychological sciences, and today it is also actively studied in neuroscience. The focus of cognitive and psychodynamic psychologists has naturally been on psychological processes rather than on brain mechanisms. However, recent experimental studies demonstrate that impaired empathy may account for the behavioral disturbances observed in both neurological and psychiatric patient populations, suggesting that empathy may be mediated by dedicated neural networks (Brothers, 1990).

Cognitive and Affective Empathy

In the broadest sense empathy refers to the reactions of one individual to the observed experiences of another (Davis, 1994). Some investigators regard empathy as a cognitive phenomenon, emphasizing the ability to engage in the cognitive process of adopting another's psychological point of view. Their research focuses on intellectual processes such as accurate perception of others (DeKosky et al., 1998). This process, which may be termed *cognitive empathy,* involves perspective taking (Eslinger, 1998) and theory of mind (Shamay-Tsoory et al., 2004), and has been reported to be dependent upon several cognitive capacities (Davis, 1994; Eslinger, 1998; Grattan et al., 1994). Other investigators have used a definition of empathy that emphasizes its affective facets. They typically study aspects such as helping behavior, and they refer to the capacity to experience affective reactions to the observed experiences of others as *affective empathy* (Davis, 1994).

The critical difference between cognitive empathy and affective or emotional empathy is that the former involves cognitive understanding of the other person's point of view whereas the latter also includes sharing of those feelings, at least at the level of gross affect (pleasant vs. unpleasant; Mehrabian & Epstein, 1972). Since it has been previously suggested that the different aspects of empathy are related and interact throughout development (Hoffman, 1978), recent theories of empathy have introduced multidimensional (Davis, 1994) and integrative (Decety & Jackson, 2004; Preston and de Waal, 2002) models that combine several aspects of empathy and empathy-related behaviors.

Corresponding to the conflicting definitions of empathy, competing theoretical views have been proposed of how we understand the behavior of others. Two different approaches attempt to account for the cognitive mechanisms that subserve the ability by which we represent and predict another person's behavior. The *theory of mind* theorists (ToM theorists) maintain that mental states attributed to other people are conceived as unobservable, theoretical posits, invoked to explain and predict behavior, something akin to a scientific theory (Gopnik & Meltzoff, 1998). According to Wellman & Wooley (1990) and other proponents of the ToM position, this kind of process is actually a "theory" of mind because beliefs and desires form the basic theoretical constructs that we combine through a system of rules to predict and explain the behaviors, thoughts, and feelings of other people.

On the other hand, the *simulation* perspective (Gallese & Goldman, 1999) emphasizes the first-person perspective and suggests that as an observer, one represents the mental states of others by tracking or matching those states with resonant states of one's own. Thus, the attributor covertly and unconsciously tries to mimic the mental activity of the target. The simulation perspective is supported by findings regarding "mirror" neurons in the monkey's ventral motor cortex that respond both when a particular action is performed by the recorded monkey and when the same action, performed by another monkey, is observed (Gallese & Goldman, 1999).

It appears that the core difference between ToM and simulation approaches to empathy is that ToM views empathy as a thoroughly "detached" theoretical analysis that involves areas of cortex that are usually activated during mental state attribution, whereas simulation depicts empathy as incorporating an attempt to replicate the other's affective mental state via neural networks related to emotion processing. With regard to the cognitive and emotional definitions of empathy, it may be suggested that cognitive empathy involves more ToM processing, whereas affective empathy involves more simulation processing.

The Neuroanatomical Basis of Empathy: The Role of the Frontal Lobes

Like many other areas of contemporary neuropsychological research, the study of empathy was first characterized by single case reports of patients suffering from brain damage. One of the first descriptions of impaired social cognition following brain damage was provided by Harlow (1868). In his famous case report, Harlow portrays the case of Phineas Gage, a railroad employee, who suffered severe frontal lobe injury from an iron bar that penetrated his frontal lobes. Although he survived, recovered physically, and had many preserved cognitive abilities, his social behavior was so impaired that his acquaintances said he was "no longer Gage." Harlow does not refer directly to Gage's empathic ability, yet he describes him as "fitful, irreverent, indulging at times in the grossest profanity, manifesting but little deference for his fellow" (Harlow, 1868).

In the following years, similar clinical reports have offered accumulating evidence regarding the role of the frontal lobes in emotion regulation and social cognition. Studies have consistently suggested that acquired damage to the prefrontal cortex may result in severe impairment in interpersonal behavior (Stuss and Benson, 1986; Damasio, Tranel, & Damasio, 1991; Stuss, Gallup, & Alexander, 2001). In particular, damage to the ventral prefrontal cortex (PFC) has been associated with misinterpretation of social situations and socially inappropriate behavior (Rolls, 1996). Eslinger and Damasio (1985) described a patient (EVR) who underwent a bilateral ablation of the orbital and lower mesial frontal cortices and, like to Phineas Gage, suffered from extensive behavioral changes. It is reported that EVR was previously successful in his professional occupation, happily married, and the father of two children. After a ventromedial (VM) prefrontal ablation, he had many difficulties in meeting his personal and professional responsibilities. He was fired from several jobs, and his wife left home after seventeen years of marriage. Despite these behavioral problems, he was described as having superior intelligence. It is reported that although he remembered social norms and had intact moral judgment, his behavior was profoundly inappropriate.

In concordance with this case, Price et al. (1990) have described two patients who suffered bilateral prefrontal damage early in life. These patients were under psychiatric attention following several incidences of aberrant behavior. A neuropsychological examination revealed deficits in moral judgment, lack of insight and foresight, impaired social judgment, impaired empathy, and difficulties in complex reasoning.

Similar evidence of impaired social cognition after early damage to the VM was reported by Anderson and colleagues (1999), who characterized the long-term consequences of early prefrontal cortex lesions in two adults who suffered prefrontal damage before they reached the age of 16 months. These patients showed impaired social behavior despite having normal basic cognitive abilities. They showed insensitivity to future consequences of decisions, defective autonomic responses to punishment contingencies, and failure to respond to behavioral interventions. However, in contrast to patients like EVR who sustained damage as adults, these patients had profound deficits in moral reasoning, suggesting that early damage to the VM region impairs social behavior as well as social perception and moral judgment.

The aforementioned case studies clearly indicate that the VM cortex mediates behaviors that involve social interactions. Although these patients' empathic abilities were never examined directly, the descriptions imply that their empathic behavior may have been impaired.

Impaired Empathic Ability Following Prefrontal Lesions

In concordance with these various definitions of empathy, several lesion studies, commencing with the work of Grattan and Eslinger (1989), have studied the empathic abilities of patients with brain damage. Grattan and Eslinger (1989) found that cognitive empathic ability was correlated with cognitive flexibility, an aspect of executive functioning that is considered to be mediated by the prefrontal cortex. These results led the authors to consider the hypothesis that impaired empathic behavior is associated with frontal lobe damage

(Grattan et al., 1994). Interestingly, they did not find significant differences in the overall self-report measure of empathic ability between patients with lesions restricted to the PFC and patients with other cortical lesions (Grattan et al. 1994). However, when the authors divided the PFC into subregions (PFC damage in the orbitofrontal, medial, and dorsolateral sections), a dissociable pattern of impairment in empathy and cognitive flexibility emerged. Apparently, impaired empathy was significantly related to cognitive flexibility in the patients with dorsolateral (DLC) damage but not in the patients in the orbitofrontal (OFC) and the medial subgroups. In the medial subgroup empathic ability was preserved while cognitive flexibility was impaired, whereas in the OFC subgroup empathic ability was impaired while cognitive flexibility was preserved. The authors concluded that impaired empathy in this group was independent of cognitive flexibility and reflected an inability to activate the appropriate somatic or autonomic states required for empathic processing.

Extending these initial efforts, my colleagues and I compared the empathic response of patients with localized lesions in the prefrontal cortex to the responses of patients with posterior cortex lesions and with those of healthy control subjects (Shamay-Tsoory et al., 2003). To illuminate the cognitive processes that underlie empathic ability, the relationships between empathy scores using the Interpersonal Reactivity Index (IRI, a self-report measure of empathic ability) and the performance on tasks that assess processes of cognitive flexibility, affect recognition, and theory of mind were also examined.

The authors reported that patients with lesions restricted to the PFC and patients with damage to the right hemisphere were significantly impaired in empathic ability as assessed using a cognitive empathy scale (the perspective-taking and fantasy subscales from the IRI). Furthermore, lesions in the VM region appeared to be associated with a greater deficit in self-reported empathy. When compared to the healthy control group, the PFC patients were impaired on the various measures of cognitive flexibility employed in this study. Of greater interest, however, was the finding that the relationships between *cognitive* empathy scores and performance on measures of cognitive flexibility, affect recognition, and ToM (assessed with the faux pas task) revealed a differential pattern in the two subgroups of PFC lesions. In the DLC group, cognitive empathic ability was related to cognitive flexibility but not to ToM, whereas in the VM group cognitive empathy was related to ToM but not to cognitive flexibility. In fact, the VM group had both the lowest self-reported cognitive empathy scores and the greatest number of errors in the ToM task. These results suggest that deficits in the ability to make an inference regarding another person's mental state may account for the lower self-reported cognitive empathy ability observed in the VM group.

In a follow-up study, we demonstrated that patients with prefrontal lesions were significantly impaired in both self-reported cognitive and affective empathy as compared to patients with parietal cortex (PC) lesions and healthy controls (Shamay-Tsoory, Tomer, et al., 2004). In order to examine whether specific regions within the PFC and the PC were associated with the mediation of affective and cognitive empathy, we divided the PFC and the PC groups into subgroups according to the exact localization of the lesion (OFC, medial PFC [mPFC], DLC). Surprisingly significant group differences were observed only for cognitive empathy but not for affective empathy, suggesting that the OFC and mPFC subgroups had significantly lower cognitive empathy scores than the PC subgroups. Additionally, the pattern of relationships between cognitive performance and empathy suggested that while cognitive empathy correlated with cognitive flexibility, affective empathy correlated with recognition of emotional facial expressions.

The Relationship between Theory of Mind and Cognitive Empathy

As mentioned above, it appears that ToM and cognitive empathic ability are closely related and depend on intact VM cortex. The neural bases of affective empathy, on the other hand, appear to be less clear. ToM is the cognitive capacity to make inferences regarding others' mental states: their knowledge, needs, intentions, and feelings (Premack & Woodruff, 1978). Indeed, it appears that cognitive empathy as opposed to affective empathy involves creating a cognitive theory of mind regarding the other's mental and emotional state. Furthermore, it has been suggested that similar brain regions participate both in cognitive empathy and in ToM. Neuroimaging studies have mainly pointed to the role of the medial prefrontal cortex in ToM. In separate studies Fletcher, Goel, and their colleagues found left medial frontal activation during performance of ToM tasks using positron emission tomography (PET; Fletcher et al. 1995; Goel et al., 1995). Using functional magnetic resonance imaging (fMRI), a similar pattern of left mPFC activation was demonstrated while participants performed story and cartoon tasks (Gallagher et al., 2000).

Gallagher and Frith (2003) have hypothesized, based on imaging studies, that the network subserving ToM includes the medial PFC, the superior temporal sulci (STS) and the temporal poles bilaterally. These authors point out, however, that while the mPFC is the distinctive key region for mentalizing, the STS and the temporal pole are not uniquely associated with ToM.

Lesion studies have similarly illustrated the role the PFC in ToM. Rowe and coworkers (2001) reported that subjects with either left or right PFC lesions are impaired in ToM ability, as assessed by first- and second-order false belief tests. Stone, Baron-Cohen, & Knight (1998) compared the performance of patients with orbitofrontal cortical damage to that of patients with dorsolateral prefrontal damage on different ToM tasks. Unlike subjects with dorsolateral damage, who performed flawlessly on all tasks, patients with orbitofrontal damage resembled individuals with Asperger syndrome, exhibiting good performance on first- and second-order false belief tasks and impairment on the faux pas task (Stone et al., 1998).

Stuss and colleagues (2001) highlighted the specific importance of the prefrontal cortex, especially the right frontal lobe and the medial PFC, in tasks of perspective taking and deception, tasks that are also considered to require ToM.

On the other hand, Bird and colleagues (2004) questioned the role of the medial PFC cortex in ToM in a recent case study. The authors described a patient, G.T., who suffered a stroke in the anterior cerebral artery territory, resulting in widespread bilateral damage to the medial PFC. While exhibiting a dysexecutive syndrome, the patient displayed intact performance on various ToM tasks such as the picture sequences, "strange story," and animation tasks. Although G.T. showed some impairment on the violation of norms and faux pas tasks, the authors concluded that this case demonstrated that the medial PFC is not essential to ToM. Samson and colleagues (2005), in agreement with Bird, recently reported evidence from brain-damaged patients showing that the left temporoparietal junction is necessary for reasoning about beliefs of others. The authors further suggested that while belief-reasoning errors of patients with PFC damage may arise from a dysexecutive syndrome, belief-reasoning errors of patients with damage to the temporoparietal junction are independent of other cognitive impairments (Samson et al., 2005).

Given this body of evidence, it appears that the exact role of the PFC cortex in ToM and its relation with empathy has yet to be elucidated. We recently suggested that the conflicting reports may reflect differences between task demands and, consequently, variation in the mentalizing processes used in these studies (Shamay-Tsoory, Tomer, et al., 2005). For example, while performance on second-order false belief tasks requires a cognitive understanding of the difference between the speaker's knowledge and that of the listener (knowledge about *beliefs*), identification of social faux pas requires, in addition, an empathic appreciation of the listener's emotional state (knowledge about *emotions*).

Using the ToM tasks devised by Stone, Baron-Cohen, and Knight (1998) and a task involving detection of irony, we previously reported that patients with lesions that involve the right VM exhibit impaired performance on the tasks that assess *affective ToM* (identifying social 'faux pas' and irony) but not on tasks which assess *cognitive ToM* (second-order false belief tasks) (Shamay-Tsoory, Tomer, et al., 2005). Moreover, examination of the relation between ToM and cognitive and affective empathy revealed a significant correlation between the poor performance of the affective ToM tasks and impaired *cognitive* empathy, suggesting that *affective* "mind reading" may, in fact, be a *cognitive* empathic response. The significant correlation between affective ToM and cognitive empathy (and the nonsignificant correlation with affective empathy) implies that although inferences of feelings and emotional experiences in other people involve affective processes, they are nonetheless still cognitive. On the basis of these results, it may be assumed that *affective* theory of mind has to do with processes of *cognitive* empathy, which are involved in the inference of other people's emotions.

The inferences one makes regarding others' mental states are based on knowledge regarding their thoughts and beliefs, as well as an empathic understanding of their emotional states and feelings. It is possible that the behavioral deficit of individuals with ventromedial PFC damage is specifically related to impairment in this affective facet of ToM and cognitive empathy, rather than to a general impairment of ToM. This idea is supported by the recent findings of Hynes, Baird, and Grafton (2006), who, using fMRI, demonstrated that the medial orbitofrontal lobe was preferentially involved in emotional as compared to cognitive perspective taking. A similar distinction between affective and cognitive ToM was made by Brothers and Ring (1992), who referred to "cold" versus "hot" aspects of ToM. Brothers and Ring further suggest that the "hot" aspects of ToM may be mediated by the medial and orbital PFC. Thus, it might be speculated that the distinct abilities for cognitive and affective mental representation involve dissociable psychological and neural mechanisms and possibly engage discrete prefrontal circuitry.

To test this hypothesis directly, we have recently developed two novel ToM tasks. The first task, illustrated in figure 16.1, is based on a task described earlier by Baron-Cohen (1995) in which participants use verbal and eye gaze direction cues to judge others' mental states. Our computerized task was designed to assess the ability to make first- and second-order affective versus cognitive mental state attributions, relying on the simple verbal and eye gaze cues and involving minimal language and executive demands. It consists of 64 trials, each showing a cartoon outline of a face (named Yoni) and four colored pictures of objects belonging to a single category (e.g., fruits, chairs) or faces, one in each corner of the computer screen. The subject's task is to point to the correct answer (the image to which Yoni is referring) based on a sentence that appears at the top of the screen and on available cues such as Yoni's eye gaze direction, Yoni's facial expression, or the eye gaze and facial expression of the face to which Yoni is referring (see figure 16.1).

No significant differences in accuracy between groups were evident in the cognitive ToM conditions and in the physical control conditions. In contrast, patients with VM damage had the most impaired performance in the affective ToM conditions. Even though all participants had better performance (high accuracy, short reaction times) in the affective ToM conditions, the VM patients appeared to show impaired performance in these conditions (Shamay-Tsoory & Aharon-Peretz, 2007).

In a follow-up study we examined the hypothesis that the VM region is important for affective ToM, using transcranial magnetic stimulation (TMS). In this study (Lev-Ran et al., submitted), 13 healthy subjects performed the same affective ToM tasks (with the drawings of Yoni) after randomly receiving low-frequency repetitive TMS (rTMS) over the VM or sham rTMS. We found that rTMS to the VM, but not sham rTMS, significantly affected processing of affective ToM stimuli. Performance on a control task, not involving affective ToM functioning, was not significantly altered after application of rTMS or sham rTMS to the VM cortex.

Based on the aforementioned neuroimaging data (Gallagher & Frith, 2003) and these lesion studies, we suggest that the cognitive and affective mentalizing abilities are controlled by a neural network that comprises the superior temporal sulci, the temporal poles, and the prefrontal cortex. Whereas basic cognitive ToM capacities may rely on the intact function of the entire network, affective ToM relies specifically on the contribution of the orbitofrontal medial region, where integration of cognitive and affective processes takes place. This suggests that individuals with VM damage are particularly impaired on tasks that

First Order	Second Order — directed toward picture	Second Order — directed straight ahead
Cognitive ToM (24 trials)		
Cog1 12 trials	Cog2 6 trials	Cog2 6 trials
Yoni is thinking of 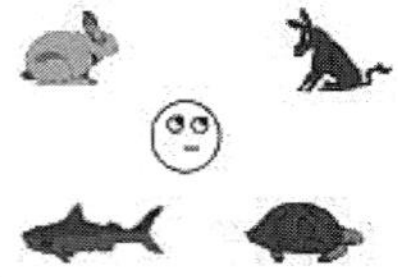 _____	Yoni is thinking of the fruit that _____ wants 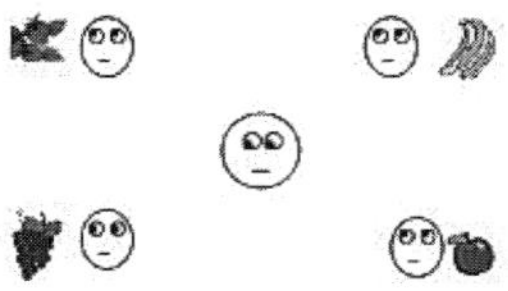	Yoni is thinking about the toy that _____ wants 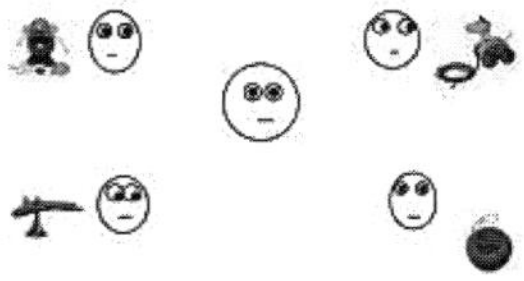
Affective ToM (24 trials)		
Aff1 12 trials	Aff2 6 trials	Aff2 6 trials
Yoni loves 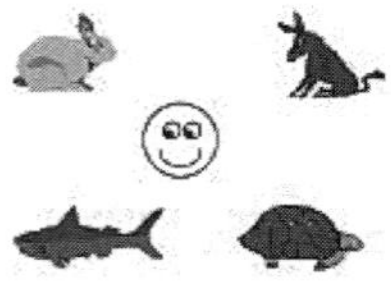 _____	Yoni loves the toy that _____ loves 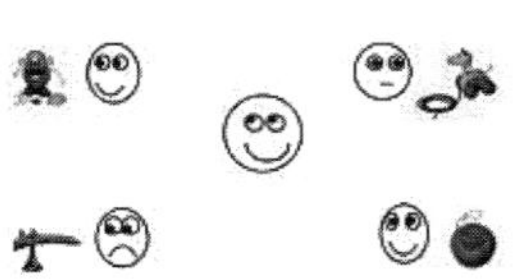	Yoni loves the toy that _____ does not love 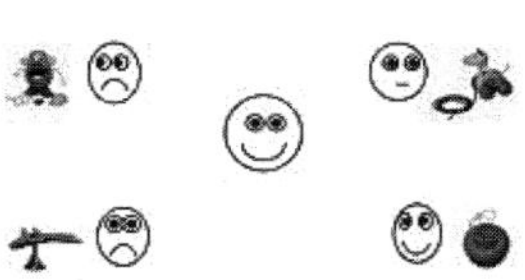
Physical Judgment (16 trials)		
Phy1 8 trials (4 directed, 4 straight ahead)	Phy2 4 trials	Phy2 4 trials
Yoni is close to 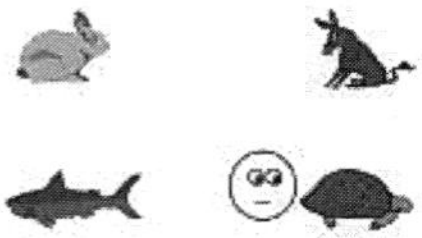 _____	Yoni has the chair that _____ has 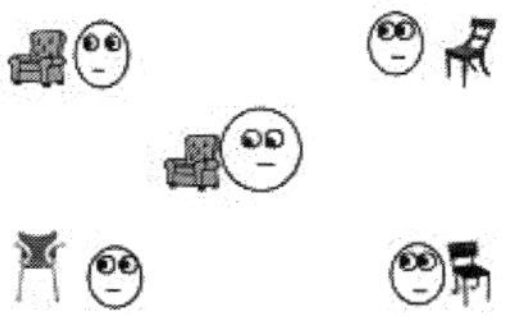	Yoni has the fruit that _____ has 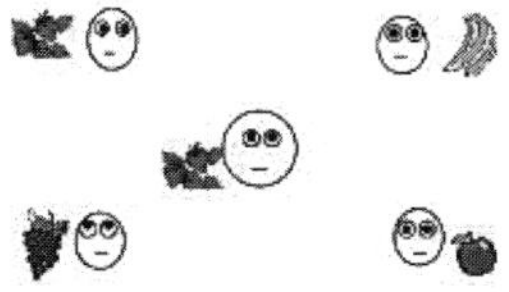

Figure 16.1

Sample of items: Cognitive and affective mental inference and a mentalistic significance of eye direction. The cognitive and affective conditions involve mental inferences, while the physical condition required a choice based on a physical attribute of the character. The cognitive, affective, and physical conditions required either a first-order (32 trials) or a second-order (32 trials) inference. In the cognitive conditions, both Yoni's facial expression and the verbal cue are emotionally neutral (Cog1), whereas in the affective conditions, both cues provide affective information (Aff1). In the second-order condition (Cog2, Aff2, Phy2), the four stimuli consist of face images and the choice of the correct response requires understanding of the interaction between each of these figures and Yoni's mental state.

involve integration of emotion and cognition, such as attribution of affective mental states (Shamay-Tsoory, Tibi-Elhanany, & Aharon-Peretz, 2006). The impairment appears to relate to the empathic abilities of these patients and, therefore, may underlie their behavioral deficits. Indeed, the intimate connections of the VM with the anterior insula, temporal pole, inferior parietal region, and amygdala place it in a position to evaluate and regulate incoming limbic information, which can consequently be used to inhibit behavior, regulate emotions, and empathize with the experiences of others.

In line with this reasoning, Mitchell, Banaji, and Macrae (2005) recently reported VM activation in a task that involves a type of affective mentalizing. In their study, subjects were asked to infer how pleased the person in a photograph seemed to be to have their photograph taken. The authors suggested that although the VM guide the understanding of others' mental states through "simulation" processing, the dorsal medial PFC may instead instantiate more generic applicable social–cognitive processes involved while mentalizing. It appears that most of the neuroimaging studies that have identified the dorsal mPFC have used very cognitive mentalizing tasks (Baron-Cohen et al., 1994; Fletcher et al., 1995; Goel et al., 1995; Gallagher et al., 2000; Vollm et al., 2006). Considering all the evidence, we may speculate that the VM mediates more affective aspects of mentalizing compared to the dorsomedial PFC.

Further Evidence for the Role of the Prefrontal Cortex in Empathy: Studies of Patients with Neurodegenerative and Psychiatric Illness

In keeping with the lesion studies reviewed above, recent evidence from studies with patients suffering from frontal lobe degeneration have supported the role of the PFC in empathy and ToM. Severe empathy loss is a common feature of frontotemporal lobar degeneration (FTLD). Lough, Gregory, and Hodges (2001) have presented the case of JM, a 47-year-old man diagnosed with frontal variant of frontotemporal dementia. JM was described as exhibiting severe antisocial behavior. His neuropsychological assessment indicated relatively intact general neuropsychological and executive function, but extremely poor performance on tasks involving theory of mind.

The neuroanatomic basis of empathy was further investigated in a large sample of patients with FTLD, Alzheimer's disease, corticobasal degeneration and progressive supranuclear palsy, using measures of self-reported cognitive empathy (taken from the IRI). Consistent with previous research implicating a primarily right frontotemporal network, empathy scores in frontotemporal dementia patients correlated with the volume of right temporal structures (Rankin et al., 2006).

Patients with schizophrenia also show impaired emotional and social behavior, such as misinterpretation of social situations, lack of empathy, and lack of ToM. It has been suggested that the neuroanatomical basis of impaired social cognition in schizophrenia involves a frontotemporal dysfunction (Lee et al., 2004). In accordance with these notions, we have recently showed that impaired affective ToM (Shamay-Tsoory, Aharon-Peretz, & Levkovitz, 2007) and cognitive empathy in schizophrenia correlates with a measure of orbitofrontal and VM(rather than dorsolateral) functioning. Furthermore, by comparing different patterns of affective and cognitive ToM impairments in schizophrenia and in patients with PFC damage, we have shown that patients with schizophrenia (particularly with negative symptoms) and those with VM lesions were impaired on affective ToM tasks (the eye gaze task) but not in cognitive ToM conditions. It was concluded that the pattern of mentalizing impairments in schizophrenia resembled that seen in patients with lesions of the frontal lobe, particularly those with VM damage, providing support for the notion of a disturbance of the frontolimbic circuits in schizophrenia (Shamay-Tsoory, Aharon-Peretz, & Levkovitz, 2007).

To further examine the dissociation between cognitive and affective ToM, we administered the eye gaze task to 13 participants with high social anxiety (HSA), 20 patients with borderline personality disorder, 17 patients with Asperger syndrome and other high-functioning adults with autism, and 20 patients with a bipolar disorder. The performance of these patients was compared to that of patients with predominantly negative or positive symptoms of schizophrenia and patients with localized lesions. As shown in figure 16.2, it appears that across all groups the correlation between cognitive ToM and affective ToM is high ($r = 0.539$) though not significant. However, dissociation between cognitive and affective ToM is apparent in the HSA and the dorsolateral PFC lesion groups. The patient group that shows the highest affective ToM is the HSA group. Indeed in this group we have also found high ratings of cognitive empathy (Tibi-Elhanany & Shamay-Tsoory, unpublished). Interestingly, these findings reveal hyperactive frontolimbic circuitry in HSA individuals (Tillfors et al., 2002), suggesting that hyperactivation of this circuit may be associated with elevated affective ToM.

Thus the aforementioned case reports, lesions experiments, and neurodegenerative and neuropsychiatric disorder studies clearly indicate that the deficit in affective ToM and cognitive empathy is associated with VM lesions rather than damage to other brain areas. However, this association should not be interpreted to mean that cognitive empathy is localized to the VM cortex. Rather, we suggest that the VM region plays a major part in a network that mediates empathy. Similarly, Brothers (1990) has described a neural circuit including the orbitofrontal cortex, the amygdala, the anterior cingulate gyrus, and the temporal pole, suggesting that this circuit functions as a unitary social "editor" specialized in the processing of others during social interaction.

A Neural Network for Cognitive and Affective Empathic Response

Considering the multifaceted nature of empathy, it is only to be expected that it would be mediated by a complex neural network involving simulation as well as mentalizing

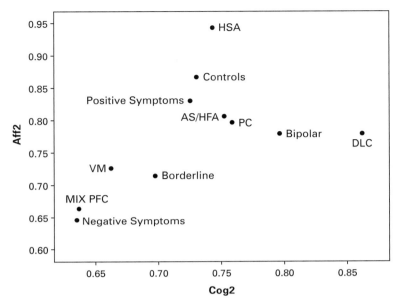

Figure 16.2
Performance in the second-order affective and cognitive ToM eye gaze task in patients with high social anxiety (HSA), controls, patients with schizophrenia with predominantly negative (Negative Symptoms) or positive symptoms (Positive Symptoms), patients with a bipolar disorder, patients with borderline personality disorder, patients with Asperger syndrome or high-functioning autism (AS/HFA), patients with posterior cortical lesions (PC), patients with ventromedial PFC lesions(VM), patients with dorso-lateral PFC lesions (DLC), and patients with VM and DLC lesions (MIX PFC).

processing. Although ToM (or mentalizing) processing has been examined extensively both in neuroimaging and lesion studies, simulation processing has been examined only in a handful of imaging studies. In line with the simulation theory, Wicker et al. (2003) reported activation in the same areas (notably the insula) previously identified as involved in the perception and production of disgust as well as during the smelling of aversive odors. These results may indicate that regions associated with the experience of emotions such as disgust can be activated by seeing the facial expression of the same emotion, an emotional empathy phenomenon described as *emotional contagion*. In concordance, Singer et al. (2004) compared brain activity while healthy volunteers experienced pain and when they observed a signal indicating that their partner was receiving a painful stimulus. The anterior insula and anterior cingulate cortex were activated in both conditions and correlated with self-reported empathy scores, whereas activations in the somatosensory cortex were seen only when participants received the painful stimulus themselves. The authors suggested that observers automatically engage in emotional empathic processes when perceiving pain in others. In line with this notion, Jackson, Rainville, and Decety (2006) have also showed that both the self's and the other's perspectives of a painful stimuli were associated with activation in the neural network involved in pain processing, including the parietal operculum, ACC, and insula. However, the self-perspective yielded higher pain ratings and involved the pain matrix more extensively in the secondary somatosensory cortex, the ACC, and the insula proper. Adopting the perspective of the other was associated with specific increases in activation of the posterior cingulate cortex and precuneus and the right temporoparietal junction. Jackson, Rainville, and Decety (2006) further suggest that pain-related activations within the ACC and insula are more posterior when a painful stimulusi is applied to the self than to others. Thus, the results reported by Wicker and colleagues (2003), Jackson, Rainville, and Decety (2006), and Singer and colleagues (2004) indicate that, in the affective empathic process, observers to some extent automatically replicate their partner's experience and a shared network is thereby activated (insula, ACC,).

In sum, it appears that although the simulation perspective may explain emotional empathic processing, ToM processes may underlie cognitive empathy. Therefore, decreased empathic response may be due to deficits in mentalizing (cognitive ToM, affective ToM) or simulation (affective empathy) processing, mediated by different neural systems (represented in figure 16.3). Although cognitive ToM may involve mentalizing of thoughts, affective ToM requires mentalizing about emotional states. Thus, while cognitive ToM is not directly involved in empathic processing, it is a prerequisite for both affective ToM and cognitive empathy.

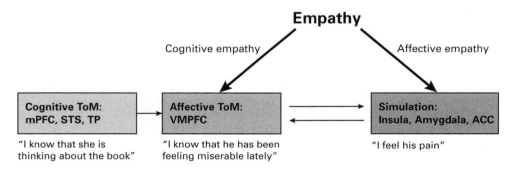

Figure 16.3
A tentative neural model of empathy. In general, the experience of empathy occurs when both the cognitive and the affective networks are activated. While theory of mind underlies cognitive empathy, simulation processing underlies affective empathy. The ToM network includes the mPFC (medial prefrontal cortex), the STS (superior temporal sulcus), the TP (temporal poles), and the VM (ventromedial prefrontal cortex). The simulation network includes the ACC (anterior cingulate cortex), the amygdala, and the insula. This network may also include the mirror neuron system (inferior frontal gyrus).